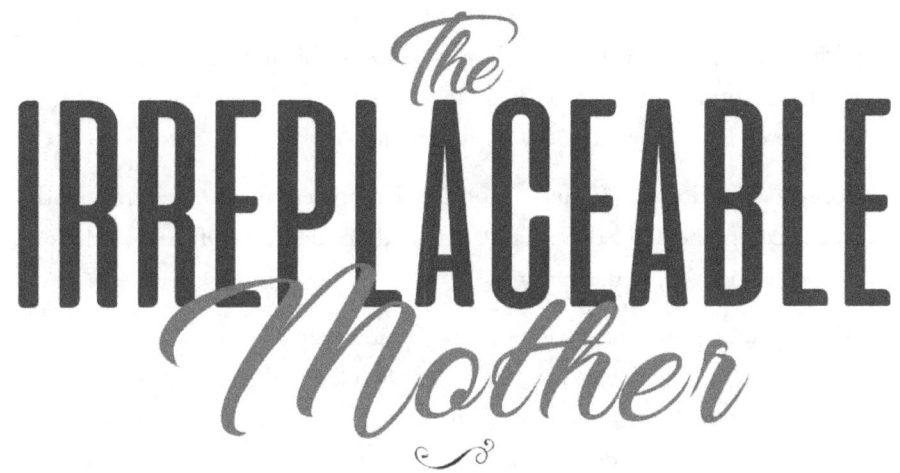

The Irreplaceable Mother

A Daughter's Journey Through
Grief and Brokenness To
Faith, Healing, and A New Normal

Lorinda Buckingham

Copyright © 2018 by Modern Empowerment, LLC, a Georgia Company

All rights reserved. No part of this publication may be reproduced, distributed, or transmitted in any form or by any means, including photocopying, recording, or other electronic or mechanical methods, without the prior written permission of the publisher, except in the case of brief quotations embodied in reviews and certain other non-commercial uses permitted by copyright law.

Lorinda Buckingham® and Modern Empowerment® are trademarks registered in the United States Patent and Trademark Office by Modern Empowerment®. All rights reserved.

All Scripture quotations, unless otherwise indicated, are taken from the Holy Bible, New International Version®, NIV®. Copyright ©1973, 1978, 1984, 2011 by Biblica, Inc.™ Used by permission of Zondervan. All rights reserved worldwide. www.zondervan.com The "NIV" and "New International Version" are trademarks registered in the United States Patent and Trademark Office by Biblica, Inc.™

Scriptures quotations marked 'ASV' are taken from the American Standard Version (1901, public domain).

Modern Empowerment books, journals, digital media, audio series, and more can be purchased in bulk for educational use. For more information, please email modernempowermentgroup@gmail.com. For free information on salvation resources, trainings, or workshops for this book email theirreplaceablemother@gmail.com.

Printed in the United States of America. All rights reserved under International Copyright Law. Contents and/or cover may not be reproduced in whole or in part in any form without the express written consent of Modern Empowerment, LLC.

DEDICATION

This book is dedicated to my Irreplaceable Mother, Ann Marie Wilson, who was the best mom, friend, teacher, role model, and confidant any of us could have ever had, and who fought a courageous battle against breast cancer. In addition, it is dedicated to all of my family, friends, and loved ones who prayed and supported me to write this book. Also, to all of those who have lost an Irreplaceable Mother, it is my prayer that you find comfort, peace, and healing in your new normal.

Scriptures

"May the God of hope fill you with all joy and peace as you trust in him, so that you may overflow with hope by the power of the Holy Spirit."
Romans 15:13

"You have turned for me my mourning into dancing; You have put off my sackcloth and clothed me with gladness, To the end that my glory may sing praise to You and not be silent. O Lord my God, I will give thanks to You forever."
Psalm 30:11-12

CONTENTS

ACKNOWLEDGEMENTS 7
INTRODUCTION 9
PROLOGUE 11

Invisible Wounds 13
   Invisible Wounds 14
   Who Is "The Irreplaceable Mother"? 29
   All Things Work Together 35

Clarity For The Grieving 41
   Grief, Mourning, and Bereavement 42
   How Do I Grieve Or Mourn? 48
   Big Boys…And Men…Do Cry 53

Overcoming Despair 57
   Is This A Bad Nightmare? 58
   I Don't Accept This! 65
   Are You Stuck In Despair? 69

Destroying Depression 73
   Destroying Depression With Faith And Prayer 74

Motherless Child In Crisis 81
   Motherless Child In Crisis 82
   Being The Strong One 86

Peace For The Abandoned And Angry 89
   It's Not Fair 90
   Hidden Anger 95
   Why Can't We Be Friends? 104

Healing Through Forgiveness 111
   Freedom With Forgiveness 112
   Forgiving Your Mother (even if she is not here) 117
   Forgiving The Elder Figures 123

Acceptance For "The New Normal" **131**
    Acceptance 132
    The "New Normal" 135

APPENDIX **139**
    What If My Mother Passed Away While I Was Young? 140
    What If I Had A Poor Relationship With My Mother? 142
    Encouragement For The Holidays 143
    Salvation (Sinners') Prayer 144
    Scriptures For Comfort 145

ABOUT THE AUTHOR 157

ACKNOWLEDGEMENTS

A special thank you to my husband, Jerome Buckingham, Jr.,
To my children,
Taylor Ann, Kendall Marie, and Jace Micah Buckingham,
And to my family and friends who supported me along the way.
And thank you to all of the people who prayed for me and encouraged me
to complete this project.

INTRODUCTION

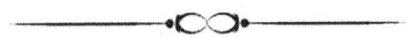

Each year in the United States, approximately 250,000 women pass away after a battle with cancer. Of those women, many have surviving sons and daughters who are left behind, struggling with grief, wrestling with unanswered questions, dealing with life drama, uncertain about their faith, and feeling stuck. They have little or no support or information to help them adjust to their new normal, of not having their mom, and that is hard.

But this book, The Irreplaceable Mother, reveals the answers that you are longing for to help you heal from the pain of loss, rekindle your hope in God, forgive those who have hurt you, and move forward in your new normal. Whether you're feeling alone, misunderstood, and submerged with many emotions, or you've processed your way through some of the darkest moments of your heart and are now wondering how to get on with your new normal, you'll find comfort, insight, and guidance from the truths uncovered in this book on how to cope with loss and pain, which I discovered through my own personal journey of grief after losing my mother to breast cancer. The empathy, relatable Christian observation, and practical principles will help your journey through grief in the healthiest, most complete way possible, so you can move forward to embrace the new life that is waiting for you.

The Irreplaceable Mother was developed from my journal entries, personal studies, and experiences to be a unique resource for motherless sons and daughters who are uncommon believers in Christ, who desire to discover how to overcome grief in a real and practical faith-based manner. In its pages, you will discover my personal journal testimony as I worked through grief, recovery, life tests and trials to achieve solace and renewed purpose in life.

Unlike what you'll find in other books, I've personally experienced the pain of loss due to the passing of my own mother after her courageous battle with breast cancer, and I've spent much time seeking answers and trying to navigate emotional, spiritual, and psychological despair. I've read and looked up many of the best books and articles on the subject of grief after losing a mother, but did not find the realness, balance, and freedom that my heart desired and faith required. Though there isn't anyone who has all of the answers, I've discovered the value of engaging in a journey to find freedom and peace after a traumatic loss and learned to be okay with my life.

Both men and women who have experienced the loss of their mom from breast cancer, pancreatic cancer, lung cancer, and other types, have already experienced encouragement, inspiration, and comfort by implementing the principles and concepts found in this helpful resource guide. Some have said, "The best thing about this book is that you can read it and begin to apply the principles in your life." Others have said that they love the down-to-earth Christian realness that is relatable and helps them pull through.

I promise that if you follow the principles in this book, you'll experience twice as much comfort, you will become inspired to live your best life, and you will enjoy many more priceless moments. And I promise that you will discover how to value yourself to have better relationships with your family and significant others.

Don't be the person who misses out on getting relief from being stuck in grief because you believe that peace and recovery are not for you. Be the kind of person other people will marvel at because of how you have changed and grown as a person. Be the kind of person who is able to say, "I remember when I used to be depressed!" "I remember when I did not want to move forward, but now I am ready to live out my legacy!" Be the kind of person who takes action and takes it immediately.

This grief resource for motherless children, no matter how young or old that you are about to read has been proven and lived out in real life. All you have to do to gain your comfort, deliverance, and freedom from grief is to keep reading. Each chapter will give you a new insight as you strive to keep time from slipping away.

Start living your life as an overcomer right now, become unstuck, and enjoy your life full of freedom, balance, and faith for success.

PROLOGUE

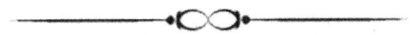

More than likely, if you are reading this book, you have either lost your mother, or you know someone who has lost a mother. Losing a mother is not an easy thing to go through. Death is a part of life, and you would think that, as many people have passed on, the subject of losing a mother would be more widely talked about. You would think that more people would have better advice to give or more comfort to provide. Yet, I find that even in this day, there are more questions and a greater lack of resources than ever before. With the increase of cancers and other sicknesses, more and more people are likely to be affected by an illness, even though life expectancy overall has increased. We see more grandmothers burying their daughters, and younger persons left without a mother. A few generations ago, it was normal to have your mother around to help you raise your children or to be around until they were old. Now because of the increase in illness, poor diets, and other external factors, having a mother around is unknown for many people.

This book was written as a mirror to the journey that I took after my mother went home to be with the Lord. As a person of faith, I found that the resources to help me to heal from my pain were very limited. I was suffering through pain, heartache, and drama, but no one really answered my heartfelt questions or dealt with the issues that I had at hand. In the midst of wanting to give up, God helped me discover how to heal. Through His word, He showed me practical ways to better understand His views about grief and loss. Throughout the process, God held me, comforted me, and showed me how to piece my life together; then He inspired me to share my discoveries with the world in hopes that it will be empowering for at least one of his many daughters and sons who have may have lost their mother.

I admit I wasn't the model Believer throughout my grief and recovery process. Which was one of the main purposes as to why I wrote this book. It was written not just for those who may know the path to take but for those who are imperfect, scarred, bruised, and broken but deep down inside love Christ. It is meant to represent those who may feel that they are forgotten, that their life is out of control, or who are unsure about where God is in the midst of their storm so that they can witness first hand an account of how down to earth God is and how He can heal them of their pain. I went through every emotion and temper tantrum that a Christian can go through after my mother passed away even doubting my faith, and yet I came back full circle to the love I originally had for Christ. That turn around was what I believed made this story remarkable. As much as I tried to leave the faith, doubted His love for me in my time of despair, and turn away from Him after experiencing the trauma I faced because of my hurt and pain, God patiently loved me and encouraged me back into relationship with Him. Not only did He bring me back 360 degrees, but the relationship between God and I became better than ever before.

In these pages, you'll find my real stories, pain, healing, practical lessons, and victory that was experienced and endured after loosing my mother to the illness of breast cancer, a person who was my best friend, the one person who 'understood me', my protector, and confidant. You will also find the word of God to help you to understand how He sees our pain and His promises about our healing. The journey of learning these lessons and writing this book was not only a fascinating one but also therapeutic in its nature. I pray that you will find this book to be refreshing, encouraging, and enlightening and that it will support you in your journey, especially if you have experienced this type of loss or are connected to someone who have experienced the loss of a mother. I also pray that it will inspire you to discover your own story, become authentic with your truth, and be unapologetic about your walk in Christ.

May God bless you in your journey of healing and coming into your new joy in your new normal.

Invisible Wounds

"Well, today I started back journaling like I did in the old days. I have always journalled, documented my life, but this time it's different... this time it's "for" my life, not just about it. I am probably in the darkest season of my life, and I don't see the light at the end of the tunnel or a pot of gold at the end of the rainbow. Right now, I am taking other people's word that this season will pass, that life will get better. I just don't know. How can things truly get better? I don't quite understand that. It's almost to say that something was wrong in the place my life used to be. My old place was my "better." The only thing that could be better is if I could have her back: safe, sound, and whole. I don't get this "better" thing.

.. I don't want the silver lining in the cloud.

I want my mom....I want her here, with us.

God, I'm lost and confused. I am hurt, angry, and afraid. This is the darkest time of my life, my family, and with me... I can't see the end of this being positive. I am so confused and sad. This life. If you desire, Lord, make me whole again. Make me free in my heart. I don't want to be angry, afraid, and confused. It seems hopeless today, God, but perhaps there's a miracle for me."

~ First Journal Entry

Invisible Wounds

My journal holds all of my secrets. Secrets that the outside world doesn't know. Secrets and thoughts that I believed that no one should know because of fear that they may judge me, criticize me, or hate me for them. What if they saw my flaws, my thoughts, and my sin? Would they put me down? The pages of my journal were like therapy and healing all in one place. They understood me and did not judge my words or criticize my thoughts. I shared them with no one, and at times not even my husband. They were all mine. But this time my journaling was different than before. I wasn't just writing about things that happened in my life or about a problem that I had. This time I was writing to *save my life*. These are my thoughts, as I had them. They are not politically correct. They don't fit into traditional religion or religious Christianity, because they are raw and real. They may not follow what most should think, but they are from my heart.

Everyone has his or her own views and perspectives. The views in this book are solely mine, based upon my own perspective and my own account of my journey, my path with my mother's health challenge with cancer, and my faith-based Christian beliefs, which are drawn from my own memory of my experiences and conversations.

After my mother passed away, there was a season where I was hurt and broken. I was unclear about my vision and lacked the motivation to succeed. I lost my sense of purpose and was uncertain about my next steps in life. Even though I was in despair, deep down inside I desired real deliverance. I desired a real healing in my soul. In my quest for healing and answers, I tried to avoid being the type of person who would assert that they had received a deliverance from a problem, but never really acquired it. Finding a middle ground that was healthy and balanced in that season of life was important to me because I desired to live happy and free without having to relinquish the love and care that I had for my mother. I came to the conclusion that would never stop missing her, but at the same time, I discovered that I needed to start the journey of learning how to live without her, which was hard.

There was a season in my journey that the grief was so difficult that I could barely speak my mother's name or about her because the pain was too deep, especially after the first year and a half after her passing. Writing this book, speaking about my journey, has not only been healing for me but has been a transporter of healing and clarity for others. I wasn't aware that on the inside that I had the strength, voice, or words to speak about my mother, yet alone my journey. Because of the depth of pain that grief can cause, my primary desire is to connect with you, as it is more important that you and I make a connection through this similar experience than for you to simply read through a concept. For a moment, I want you to give yourself permission to draw from my journey complimentary occurrences to find your own voice, words, and power to obtain healing in your own life. Sharing my journal, my life experience, and having a platform to be authentic with others has charged my soul with life and freedom. I'd be the first to admit that being vulnerable wasn't one of my strongest qualities, but yet I felt emboldened and confident in sharing my emotions, my inner thoughts, and my pain, so that it will inspire a person in their darkest hour to walk towards freedom, encourage or establish their faith in Christ, and empower them to live in joy in their new normal in the great memory of their mother after they have passed away.

In addition, I hope that my depiction of the realities that I encountered during my mother's battle with cancer and the grief recovery process will bring a level of realness and comfort to a person who is hurting. During the times of grief, our Comforter is the Holy Spirit. We can see this in the passage of scripture in the bible from the book of John:

> *"And I will pray the Father, and he shall give you another*
> *Comforter, that he may abide with you forever."*
> *John 14:16 (ASV)*

The word 'comfort' means to ease someone's grief or distress or to console. The Holy Spirit gives us comfort and eases our grief. It is refreshing to know that He abides or lives with us. He is right there with us when we are in our darkest hour. This is so refreshing because we know by faith that we are not alone.

Wounded Warrior

I was wounded after my mother passed away because I was hurt by the loss. I had taken a hard hit to my soul and felt as though was struck with a devastating blow to the heart. When I finally realized my mother was no long with me, I didn't know what hit me. You or someone you know may feel or have felt the same way. The experience of the loss can feel like a delayed reaction or a fast sharp wound acquired in a battle or fight. In that instance, it could have felt as though you have lost in life and there is no hope. However, it does not mean that you have lost at anything or are without hope. It means that a life-changing event has occurred and that you are or have transitioned into a new season of life that will require you to step into your faith, confidence, and hope as a warrior. So who is a wounded warrior? Wounded warriors are courageous individuals who have discovered they are not invincible or immortal, and have accepted that their heroism is defined not by not getting hurt but by the fact that they were willing to get into the fight.

I encourage you to give yourself grace if you have been wounded. By facing your fears, and taking on this new challenge and season of life, you are demonstrating that you are willing to take hold of the victory.

In order to take hold of the victory and get through grief, we must develop a prayer life. Our prayer life is what will carry us through the hard times, help us gain clarity, and declare our victory in times of war against the attacks of our opponent called the devil, who is thief that is always seeking to steal, kill, and destroy. His attacks include but not limited to stealing our peace, joy, and clarity.

> *"The thief comes only to steal and kill and destroy; I have come that they may have life, and have it to the full."*
> *John 10: 10*

I'm not a veteran trained by the military, but I view our prayer lives as a way for us to go into war. Prayer is a tactic that we can use after we have been wounded with grief after the loss of a loved one. Our prayers, confessions, scriptures, and worship are what we use for battle. I believe that prayer is not just monologue, where we are simply speaking to God in one-sided communication, but its *dialogue* between God and us. During our prayer time in times of grief, we get the opportunity to engage in a relationship with Him through worship, praise, and our words. We declare war against distressing emotions and situations that steal, kill, and destroy our hopes and positive aspirations. We prepare for our victory, share our concerns, get recharged, gain clarity, and so much more during prayer.

After learning about prayer in a bible study group, I was hooked. I tried to pray often. I was known to enjoy and love prayer. However, there was a moment where I lost the desire to pray in my prayer life after my mother passed way. It was hard for me to find my voice and the words to pray because I was hurting. Instead of being the faith-filled prayer warrior soldier that I had learned to become in the bible study group, I was acting more like a wounded puppy. I lost the zeal and heart to pray like I used to. I had been trained in church on how to pray, attended small groups, and have worked in ministry, but in that season of my life, I was almost speechless. My prayer life started to slip slowly but surely. I was trying to force myself do something that was once so easy and joyful to do. Perhaps you or someone you know could relate to that pain and the struggles with maintaining a prayer life after a major loss. If you notice in my journal entry above, I was in despair. Yet, at the end of that entry, I was still holding on for a miracle. I was hurting, but deep down on the inside of my heart, I wanted God to save me. I know that there are many who can relate. They are hurt and unable to pray, but deep down inside they desire for God to save them from their despair.

Even though I was wounded, my wounds were unseen because they were under a mask. I put on a mask and wore it every day to cover up my true condition of hurt, anger, and grief. I wore it in an effort to deny and dismiss my reality in fear of failure, judgment, and the ridicule of others. I did not want to hear from others about what I should do or feel. I just wanted to be heard and respected for what I was feeling and experiencing at the time without judgment or prejudice.

For me, the wounds that I experienced from losing a mother to cancer took me off balance because of the long journey of doctor appointments, chemo treatments, special diets, and medical bills. Dealing with medical emergencies and issues can cause our equilibrium to get off track. The good news is that wounded soldiers have promises that they will receive the clarity, deliverance, and healing that they need.

During combat, despite being wounded, a soldier must pull through to get to safety and to the medic. If you are wounded, like I was, you will have to make a decision to be intentional about getting to the Healer and to receive your healing. I'd like to envision that when a Christian is in troubled times and in need of help that our healing assistance is similar to that of when a rescue helicopter comes in to lift troops out of a troubled situation during war. In Christ, I believe that our rescue helicopter that is always ready to help us is called the Holy Spirit, who is also called our Helper. The Holy Spirit is ready to supply healing, restoration, and comfort, and lifts us out of danger, despair, depression, and heal us of our wounds. As mentioned, our wounds are merely indicators that we have been hurt and that we need re-adjust our lives to manage our injuries, but it does not have to hinder us from living a happy and productive life. I want to encourage you, that if you need help through a season of loosing a mother to seek the help of God and to reach out to other like-minded soldiers who are strong in faith and can support you without judgment to help get you to the other side of your grief.

Painful Realities

My mother has gone home to be with the Lord, and I don't know what to do. How do I move on? I still needed her. I have more questions that I need to have answered. Who will help me through all of my issues and give me advice? Like many, I had many questions and wanted answers. I could not see how to get out of the hole that I was in because I could not see the big picture.

It was hard for me to see that picture because it was wrapped up in my personal story that began a few years prior to discovering my mother's illness. My life appeared to have been going in the right direction. I graduated from high school and started my college journey at Tuskegee University to study electrical engineering. I had big dreams of graduating, becoming an engineer, working an exciting job, getting married, and living a great life.

The Irreplaceable Mother

During my time in undergrad, I grew in my faith and was very active in local churches and campus ministries. Initially, I was very shy about being involved in church because I did not feel that I fit in with organized church. I loved Christ, but my life circumstances were very complicated. I learned so much from them during that time. I held small group bible studies in the basement of my dorm building called Adams Hall, did door-to-door evangelism, and had weekly Bible studies on campus. I had great friends and a great church.

To my pleasant surprise, I discovered that there were people who were just like me in church! Because I did not come from a church background, I always felt a little out of place or like an underdog because I had a lot of flaws and did not fit into the stereotypical picture of the "perfect Christian." Initially, I did not think many people would like me because of my background, problems, and down-to-earth style. However, my Pastors, First Lady's, spiritual fathers, spiritual mothers, and brothers & sisters in Christ that loved me, always encouraged me to be authentic because they said that God will use it one day.

I was heavily involved in ministry in college, so much so that I had taken some time out of college after my junior year at Tuskegee to attend Rhema Bible Training Center in Tulsa, OK to study youth ministry. After graduating from Rhema, I went back to Tuskegee to complete the last portion of my electrical engineering program. At the time, I did not have the support of my family to leave school or to be a part of the ministry. First, it was because they did not want me to leave college and take the risk of dropping out of school. Second, they did not share the same commitment and understanding of my faith as I did and therefore did not understand the value or discernment to follow a God-inspired direction. I understood some of their concerns and opposition to my decision as it related to my education but I had a strong leading in my spirit to discover how to better serve God and His people. I did not take my decision lightly. I prayed, fasted, and received counsel for months before making my final decision to leave college in Alabama and to move to Bible College in Oklahoma. I also knew that my family and I were not on the same page or trajectory of faith and would not be able to understand or connect to the journey or decision that I was on. I admit was a huge risk to make the decision to follow the leading of the Holy Spirit at the tender age of 20 years old to leave college to go to bible school, and not so much to become an ordained minister but to get training on how to develop the skill set to help equip leaders, youth, and individuals to become better in their lives. It definitely wasn't my idea. It was a vision that I believe that God gave me and was in my heart. While I attended Rhema Bible Training Center, all of my needs were met, and I had an amazing two years of school learning how to serve in local ministries, individuals, youth, and non-profit organizations.

After graduating from Rhema, I went back to Tuskegee to complete my engineering program. I thought at the time that my life was on the same track. I did not know this at the time, but the types of decisions to follow the Holy Spirit or follow my faith would later pose problems within some of my family dynamic and friend circles when my mother passed away because each of us were going down different paths of faith and life. I was making decisions that were placing me on the outside and separating me from the rest of my family and friends that I was not aware of.

Upon returning to Alabama to finish my degree at Tuskegee, I interviewed and offered an opportunity to work on staff as a Campus Minister for a church named Word Of Faith in Birmingham, AL to do campus ministry at Tuskegee and youth ministry support for the church; where I would conduct small groups, women's and girls' bible studies, and more. I also volunteered with the Tuskegee Student Government Association (SGA), advising on spiritual affairs. I had high hopes and ambitions after graduating from college of living a so-called 'perfect life.' I had a diverse group of friends, and I felt as though I was headed down the right path in my education and faith. After graduating from college with a bachelor's degree in electrical engineering, I started preparing for a new career in the automotive industry as an engineer after graduation.

During the course of my career, I met and married my husband. He was also a born-again Christian, believed in the Bible, was in the engineering industry, and was as fun-loving as I was. My husband and I were young, free, and in love. I don't think I ever knew that I could love a man so deeply. He was not only a man of faith, but he valued me as a woman to respect me as both my *Father's* and my *father's* daughter. In my eyes, we were headed towards the perfect happily ever after, because we were nice Christian people and therefore in my mind it meant that we would have a good life without any issues or complications. I soon discovered that I had created a common yet unhealthy fairy-tale life, and had developed expectations about myself, my marriage, and my life that were setting me up for heartbreak and disappointment. Ultimately those relationship and life expectations were going to play a role in how well I was going to handle and move forward in my journey of grief recovery after my mother passed away from cancer. Little did I know, that these types of unhealthy expectations would put stress on a relationship and marriage after her passing.

After a few years of marriage, my husband and I began to start a family. We were excited to be parents! Both of our families were excited when we shared the news about our first child. The moment was surreal. Jokingly, my husband and I remember when I was standing in the mirror, and I said that I did not look pregnant or feel pregnant, but the pregnancy test said that I was. Our family and friends teased that I would soon see the difference and that I would be making a transition to elastic pants.

I remember the look on my mother's face when she learned that she was going to be a grandmother. She was so proud and happy. She couldn't wait to tell all of her girl friends and colleagues at work that she would be joining the ranks of grandparents. She decided that she wanted to be called "NaNa." She decided that she was too cool to be called grandma and that she was going to be a stylish grandmother. We all loved witnessing her enjoy her moment. You could see the joy beam off of her face and happiness radiate from her eyes. My mother began to schedule time off work even though my due date was about eight and a half months away. Her excitement spilled over as to sound the alarm to all of the women that she will be joining the ranks of being a grandmother and it was what she had been waiting for.

But things began to change…

During the last month of my pregnancy, as we were preparing for the baby's arrival, my mother became ill. I noticed that she would become sleepy or tired as we were shopping for baby furniture or clothes. I thought she had a cold or was tired from the hours she worked. She was known to work extra hours and to cover for people if they needed time off work. She tried to push through it, but I could tell it was a lot. I made up excuses about being tired to end our trips early. I tried not to bother her with anything about the baby. Secretly, I was disappointed because I wanted to experience the mother-daughter moments of having a baby, but I did not want to push it or make it all about me if my mother had a cold or the flu. Plus, I figured she needed to rest up to prepare to help me after I had the baby and we can make up for the time later. Yet, my mother's cold continued to linger.

My mother went to the doctor a few times about not feeling well. I did not think much of it. In the past, she would take medications, and move on. As time drew in closer to the birth, there was a lot of excitement amongst the family about the arrival of the new baby.

When I gave birth to my husband and I first-born daughter in January 2010, we were the happiest and proudest parents. Everyone flooded the hospital and wanted to take pictures of the baby. I was exhausted from the delivery and did not care about how I looked. To know my mother is to know that she was the type of woman who valued fashion and make-up. Before taking pictures, my mother insisted that I put on a little make-up and some lipstick to take my first family and baby pictures in the hospital. It was a comical experience because she acted as though make-up and lipstick were the cure to everything. It was one of our fondest memories of her. We likened her to the dad who played Gus, in the movie *My Big Fat Wedding*, who used Windex to solve every illness and problem. We were all humorously convinced that our Trinidad and Tobago mother would get cast to play in the sequel, but this time use lipstick to solve every illness and problem.

After being discharged from the hospital, I returned to the comfort of my home. My mother came over that day, after a doctor's appointment, to help me get situated with the baby. Throughout the day, she was unusually solemn and quiet. I asked her if everything was okay; she said yes. Yet, she seemed so distant. There would be a rare moment of liveliness whenever she held the baby, but she kept to herself for the most part.

My mother continued to help me with getting around and with the baby for a few days but was still distant. My husband was very attentive and helping a lot. She spent a few days with me, but she did not talk much or was as comical as before. I started to worry that something was wrong because it was not normal for her. Typically, I would push the issue, but I was so tired from the delivery and recovery that I did not have much energy to ask anymore questions.

However, about a month or so later, I asked her again what was on her mind and why she was acting so distant. My mother shared with me that the doctors had found something in her breast--a lump, but she said that it was not that big of a deal and that she would be okay. I was shocked and unclear about the words that I was hearing. It was like I was hearing words from a slow motion promo video. My mother further explained that she had found out about it around the time that I was about to have the baby following a series of tests. My heart sank to the floor.

This was a painful reality for me.

As the oldest daughter, I immediately jumped into protective mode and asked why she hadn't said anything sooner. She said that she didn't tell me the truth because she did not want to worry me. She wanted me to focus on having my first baby and enjoying the happy moment of becoming a mother. I stared at her with mixed emotions and a look of bewilderment on my face. I did not know what to feel or say in that moment. One on side, I was angry with her, but on the other side as a new mother, I understood some of her perspectives.

What is happening to my mother and to our family? I thought. *"Will she be okay? How is she taking this?"* This season of life was supposed to be one of the happiest seasons of all where I enjoy the moments of parenthood with my husband, my family, and my mother. While recovering from welcoming a new life in our family, simultaneously I was faced with the possibility of the exit of another's life: my mother, and one of my best friends, and that was hard.

I was overwhelmed with learning how to be a new mother and all of the responsibilities that come with it. My husband and I enjoyed being parents because our daughter was like a ray of sunshine and joy in our lives. We couldn't have felt more blessed. At the same time, I was feeling so unlucky and cheated because I was also worrying about my own mother and her illness. I felt as though my mother was being robbed of being a grandmother, that all of us would not have the experience of having a mother with us when we gave birth and raised our children. Not forgetting, what other experiences that other members in the family may have felt that they may have lost. On the inside, I felt like I was having an internal meltdown. The entire time I thought she had just had a cold; then I learned that it was more and that she had gone to the doctor for something more serious.

The thought of raising my children without the support of my mother was scary, and I did not want to entertain it at the time. I decided to do my best to stay focused on the positive things and do my best to overcome the current situation in front of me.

Growing Pains

My husband and I had only been married for about three and a half years when the news of my mother's illness was announced to the immediate family. My marriage was still in its young stages. The stress of work, a new baby, a young marriage, and a sick mother was taking its toll on our relationship. The honeymoon phase had faded away, and marriage realities had set in. My husband and I did our best to work together during that season, but we struggled with how to navigate through all of our life-changing events as a couple. Our communication and connection were strained. We both misunderstood each other and were on autopilot in our relationship. Neither one of us were prepared for what we were facing. Both my husband and I are the first-born children in our families and were usually the ones who took care of everyone else. Therefore, it was hard for us to get support from family members in times that we needed. Reflecting back, our challenges were not because he wasn't a good husband or I wasn't a good wife; rather because neither one of us knew how to go through tough times together or knew how to respect each other's truth. We didn't know how to connect to each other's pain, especially when there were multiple problems. We could only see our individual needs and desires at the time. There were so many moving pieces, that it felt that when it rained it poured. In that season, we had to learn how to respect each other's truth as it related to what we were experiencing at the time, pray with each other, connect with each other, and fight for our marriage. It was not just about us, but also about our family. We did not know what we were doing. We only knew that based upon our Christian beliefs that our marriage was not a contract but a covenant, and that we loved each other.

"Is love enough?" we wondered. I tend to think that love is a good step in the right direction, but it takes a little more. It takes a combination of love, forgiveness, respect, prayer, faith, intimacy, patience, and accountability to live out the Word of God to make it through times of sickness, grief, and loss. I believe that when a married couple deals with major life-changing issues in their relationship such as cancer, grief, or loss especially in the early years of marriage, it rapidly matures or ages the relationship. It the early years of a marriage, a couple is still learning each other as husband and wife. However, it does not matter what season or how long a couple may have been married: dealing with a life-changing event such as cancer or any illness can add stress to even the so-called best marriages.

My husband and I believed in the fact that that marriage is a covenant and that love is an action word. We loved each other, but we had to discover how to do life together as friends and lovers in that tough season. It was hard to work through those tough moments but possible through faith.

What should you do if you or someone you know is having a tough time in their marriage or relationship after loosing a mother to cancer and dealing with grief? Have patience! Have faith! Faith for a better day! Have faith in a brighter future, understanding about each other, and clarity about your vision as a couple together. I am learning that the source of discord in marriages when dealing with traumatic situations isn't always the issue itself, but it is how the couple responds to each other during those troubling times. Discovering how to become selfless, giving up the need to be right, and sincerely respecting each other for who they are and their truth, will help a married couple get to the other side of the trouble patch in their marriage.

By the grace of God, we were able to get to the other side stronger than ever, but it wasn't without prayer, grace, and work. I want to encourage you, if you are having a hard time in your marriage or relationship with a significant other during your time of bereavement, to hold on and allow the fog to clear before making any rash decisions about your relationship. Pray to God. Ask for His help to discover how to deal with loss as a couple, especially if there are children involved. There are no guarantees that a relationship will work or last. Maintaining a relationship takes effort.

Christian marriages have issues just like everyone else's. If anything, a Christian couple or a couple of faith-based values may endure many attacks on their relationship because our enemy, the devil, hates marriages. Marriage is the one thing that resembles Christ and the church. This is shown in the scripture below:

> *"'For this reason a man will leave his father and mother and be united to his wife, and the two will become one flesh.' This is a profound mystery—but I am talking about Christ and the church."*
> *Ephesians 5:31-32*

Our marriages and relationships have a greater purpose. Most people do not go into a relationship expecting it to fail. I cannot say whether a person should stay or not in their marriage or relationship, but I would offer that if a person is going through a traumatic time of loss of a mother, that if possible, to allow some time to pass so that they can see how to successfully navigate through their marriage and decisions.

Remember, you are not alone, and you can do this! Believe God for clarity and direction to guide your path to healing, restoration, and recovery for your marriage and family.

Healing Your Unseen Wounds

Healing the wounds that are unseen takes determination and courage. You may find yourselves reluctant to work towards the promise of healing after the passing of a mother because we have lived without your healing for so long. After reading this section, you may realize that you have wounds that you were not aware of that requires your attention. Most importantly, you may be motivated to take action towards the life that you desire. Witnessing my mother's life example has inspired me to live my best life, and, when the time comes, to die my best death. To live our best life, means we must decide to get clear on our purpose, passion, vision, and do the work necessary to achieve success. To die our best death means to have faith in where you are going. It reminds me of when the Apostle Paul said,

"For to me, to live is Christ, and to die is gain."
Philippians 1:21

My mother had faith about where she was going. I have faith in where I am going. If you do not have faith in where you are going, there is a prayer in the back of this book that you can pray so that you can start living as a child of God in confidence. When you make the decision to surrender your life to Christ and to live your best life, you are on the road to recovery from the loss of a mother.

By taking these steps, you are starting the journey of recovery by being open-minded, acknowledging your wounds, receiving the promise of the Holy Spirit's comfort, and taking steps live intentionally. It also means that you have welcomed the opportunity to learn something different, receive something new, and to learn how to live victoriously.

When you accept Christ into you heart, you belong to God. God loves you. He will never leave you nor forsake you. There is not a need to wallow in self-pity, but to renew your mind to have hope for a brighter day and future.

Here is a great scripture to reference that:

"Do not conform to the pattern of this world, but be transformed by the renewing of your mind. Then you will be able to test and approve what God's will is—his good, pleasing and perfect will."
Romans 12:2

Therefore, as you identify your invisible wounds and go through the healing process of grief recovery, be willing to have an open mind to what God will teach, expose, and heal within you during in this journey.

In the next chapters, we will uncover more foundational principles that start the process of healing. Be patient and encouraged during your course of self-awareness as you discover how to turn your pain into purpose. Many of your wounds that were unnoticed may become more visible. Our initial instinct is to run away from them to ignore them in hopes that they will go away. I encourage you to avoid that choice but to make the decision to face the hard truths in your life and your story in hopes to gain a better sense of reality and life. Get ready to get noticed. Not so much by others, but to be able to recognize the truth and power within yourself. It may seem as though you will never be able to dig your way out of the pit of despair. Many others have gone before you and have made it to the other side. You too will experience the freedom and wholeness that you desire. By faith and patience with intentional actions, you will overcome despair and find your joy and happiness once again.

Invisible Wounds
Making It Personal

Do you have any Invisible Wounds? If so, what are they? What challenges do you see that could hinder you from healing your wounds? How do you think your life would change if you were healed of your wounds? What actions could you take to start living your best life?

Who Is "The Irreplaceable Mother"?

"There isn't anyone who is like her. I miss her. Now that she's gone, people act as though they can do anything they want with me or say anything to me.
I am not going to let anybody make me feel guilty because I wanted to take time for myself and needed to use my energy to focus on being a mother to my children. My mother was one of a kind and she would be here to help me. In my heart, she was my mother not just because of her title but because she loved me.

~ Journal Entry

Who Can I Call A Mother?

The subject of mother and respect is always complicated. Once a mother or matriarch passes away, chaos can break loose. I will share more about that later. First, let's talk about the definition of Irreplaceable. In order to really understand the depth of pain or despair a person may feel once their mother passes away, we must understand the potential value of their mother. Here is a definition that I use for irreplaceable:

Irreplaceable means unique, one of a kind, no substitute, and incapable of being replaced. Priceless.

During the time of grief, we can have peace in knowing that we were fortunate enough to experience a relationship with a person who is valued, priceless, having no substitute, and who is one of a kind. Our initial reaction to the loss of a mother can vary from person to person. In each case, it's good to celebrate her uniqueness and one-of-a-kind qualities that you loved dearly.

For example, the Mona Lisa is considered one of the most valuable and priceless works of art in the world. It's considered "irreplaceable." Many of us may have our own words that describe our mother as it relates to being irreplaceable such as priceless, the cream of the crop, top notch, one in a million, our favorite girl, best friend, confidant, and irreplaceable. The list can go on and on. A mother is the person who resonates within you as being that mother figure to you.

People have various types of relationships with their mother. Depending on the relationship with the mother that has passed away, will determine how a person will respond to her passing. Regardless of what type of relationship you may have had with your mother, one of her destiny-fulfilling moments was bringing you into this world. You have a purpose and a great plan for your life. In the book of Jeremiah, it says:

"...For I know the plans I have for you," declares the LORD, "plans to prosper you and not to harm you, plans to give you hope and a future..."
Jeremiah 29:11

This passage of scripture is refreshing because it declares that God has plans to give you hope and a future. Your future is bright even if in this season it appears dark. You have a chance to do something different in your life, with your children, and redesign your future according to your destiny. Remember, a mother is valuable because she is one of a kind. The *type of value* is determined by the way she led her life with you and the experiences you believe that you shared. From the beginning, when we were in our mother's womb, our heavenly Father loved us and called us blessed.

"For you created my inmost being; you knit me together in my mother's womb.
I praise you because I am fearfully and wonderfully made..."
Psalm 139:13-14

God took His time to form you inside your mother's womb. The type of relationship we had with our mothers, whether poor, non-existent or otherwise, does not affect our identity in Christ or our ability to receive healing in the time of grief. Our self-value and self-worth are not based upon what our parents say or don't say, or the decisions that they made or don't make. In Christ, we have a new DNA and become a part of God's family as children of God. In a familiar, comforting passage of scripture, John describes this to us:

The Irreplaceable Mother

*"Yet to all who did receive him, to those who believed in his name,
he gave the right to become children of God..."*
John 1:12

I love how this passage says "all." It does not say "some." Therefore, our self-value and self-worth in this process are not based upon our mother's works or whether or not we got along with her. We can receive it if we believe on His name. Therefore, avoid the trap of guilt or condemnation during this process of healing if your relationship with your mother during her life were less than favorable. Whether the relationship was good, bad, or non-existent, our relationship with God is always available to us if we choose it.

The definition of a mother is not limited to the woman who physically gives birth to a child. A mother is defined by more than biological childbirth. A mother could be the person that you view as or who resonates as being a mother *to you*. I personally believe that it is possible to have more than one mother figure as long as you are comfortable.

There may be instances where people may try to assert themselves as mother figures after your mother's passing. I personally believe that it is not required to treat anyone as though they are your "mother" unless you are comfortable and that they resonate in your heart as a mother figure.

Biological and Adoptive Mothers

The term "birth mother" is often referred to as the mother who physically gave birth to the child. The term "adoptive mother" is often referred to as the mother who takes a child into her family by choice and assumes the role of mother to love and raise that child. The adoptive mother is the child's mother. Giving biological birth to a child is not the only pathway to being considered "the mother." Once a child is adopted, his or her adoptive mother also becomes their mother. If you have been adopted or were raised by another figure, the choice is yours on how you would deal with "the mother" question. You should be comfortable with and respectful to all parties with your decisions but live out your truth.

The best way to get clarity on how to handle these types of decisions is with prayer and counsel. If you are in a season where you are dealing with grief because the person that you identify with as 'mother' has passed away then there may be a need for closure and healing regardless of whether the person is considered the birth mother or an adoptive mother. A mother, whether she is biological or adoptive, is not "like" your mother—she *is* your mother. In the teaching of Christ, we learn that those who have accepted Christ in their hearts and lives are also adopted into the family of God. We know this to be true because of the passage of scripture that says:

> *"...He predestined us for adoption to sonship through Jesus Christ, in accordance with his pleasure and will..."*
> *Ephesians 1:5*

For all of those who have placed their faith in Christ, they have been adopted as children into the family of God our Father. Because they have been adopted into the family of God, they receive all of the blessings and benefits that come with the adoption such as forgiveness, acceptance, righteousness, and becoming a brand new creature in Christ, just to name a few. In the same way, when a person adopts a child into their family, that child gets all of the benefits of the family.

Foster Care and Caregiver Mothers

A person who takes care of you through foster care or is a caregiver can be considered a mother. For example, a grandmother, an aunt, a church mother, or whoever has taken on the responsibility to love, care for, and cherish you as their child, and impart positive things to you, is a mother or a mother figure to you. A foster parent or caregiver can play a valuable role in a person's life as a mother figure because they may have filled in the gaps in your life when it was needed. If that person resonates as a mother figure in your heart, then you can embrace them that way.

Surviving Parent's Significant Other

Your living parent may or may not have a spouse or significant other. You are free to have healthy relationships with others based upon how those relationships resonate with your heart and how comfortable you are about the situation. The best thing to do is to express how you feel and what your boundaries are. If you desire to have that relationship with your significant other's family, then set out the steps for how someone can do that with you and allow them to be there for you. If you are not interested, express that you are not interested. Most importantly, choose to be healthy and walk in your truth.

Mother-In-Law Or Stepmother-In-Law

It is very common for a mother-in-law or stepmother-in-law to step in and give support in times of bereavement or to help fill in the gaps for men and women. It is very honorable and is usually typical protocol. If you desire the assistance and it is helpful, it can help in your journey of grief recovery. On the other hand, if it makes you feel uncomfortable to have anyone else around, then you have the right to be honest about your feelings, and they should be respected. Sometimes, this may be difficult because it may be your significant other's mother. However, you are not required to treat her as your mother in the same manner as you did your own if you did not or do not have a relationship with her. To ensure that you are on the right path, be sure to pray and seek guidance on how to handle your specific situation.

It will be great if you can build an affectionate friendship with your mother in law or significant other's mother figure. If she is genuinely trying to have a good relationship and respects your boundaries, then you can create a relationship with her, as you are comfortable. However, if it makes you uncomfortable, sad, or if you simply need space, be sure to communicate that. Be sure to communicate clearly and with love to your spouse or significant other what your needs are, and your boundaries. Try to have an open and honest dialogue and continue to move towards your healing. This is the time to try to get your healing in a healthy and positive way.

Stepping In

Surviving family members and close friends should make themselves and their resources available to children and young adults. Be open to speaking about the deceased mother, going to the funeral site, celebrating special traditions, and filling in the gaps when needed. Be mindful of their milestones, ask them if they need help and offer it when it's needed. Children may not come to you directly. They may look to see what you will say or do. Allow them to be themselves. Allow them to be okay and at time not feeling up to par. The child may not have processed their situation entirely. Remember, they are working through things too.

Sometimes just bringing someone to help out with a child could help the grief recovery process. For example, tell them that someone will take them out for the day, help with a special project, or special event. Simply try to be present in their lives. If you do not have a support system or people who can provide that, then do the best you can. Once a mother passes away, many people do not know how to cope after the funeral. It is easy to leave the funeral and ignore the fact that there may have been young adults or children left behind without a mother. If the mother that has passed had young children, try to remember to check in on their children to make sure that they are okay.

During this time we have to learn how to function in a new normal, be open about our feelings, and get the support we need to move forward.

Who Is "The Irreplaceable Mother"? Making It Personal

What does it mean to you to be an Irreplaceable Mother? Who do you identify with as being your Irreplaceable Mother? What are the best things about your Irreplaceable Mother that makes her irreplaceable, priceless, and one of a kind?

All Things Work Together

> *"I'm a woman of faith and have lost one of the most precious persons to me, my mom.*
> *My faith in Christ must keep me. It is all that I have. It is all that could possibly save me. I am starting to believe that in great loss and suffering there's opportunity to grow in a deeper relationship with Christ. I'm learning that it is easy to serve him when everything goes your way, but what about when it does not?"*
> ~ *Journal Entry*

Feeling Forgotten

It is not uncommon to feel lost, confused, or forgotten after the passing of a loved one.

The passing of my mother was not any different. When my mother passed away, it was the hardest experience of my life. At times, I wanted to give up. I felt alone, and I felt out of touch with church. I was a woman in crisis. The road seemed dark because I had lost one of my best friends and the person who knew me and loved me the best.

After my mother passed away, I felt forgotten because I had lost a main person who was mindful of me. My mother thought about my well-being daily and contacted me regularly. After she passed away, I felt as though I lost that one person who was concerned about me without wanting anything in return. I no longer received the little phone call or text message to check in to see how I was doing, that came from my mother. From that experience, I had to learn how to become more empowered in my new truth. I embraced a truth that I will always miss my mother and that I was not forgotten. I did not see it at the time, but the pain of feeling forgotten had a purpose. God was not done with me yet, and He is not done with you. It reminds of me of the passage of scripture that says,

> *"And we know that in all things God works for the good of those who love him, who have been called according to his purpose."*
> *Romans 8:28*

It didn't say that it was necessarily going to feel good, but it says that all things—not some—work together *for good* to those who love God. Our emotions may tell us that we are forgotten because we are no longer getting the phone calls or text messages from our mother like we were in the past. I encourage you to hold on to the same promise, that even if it doesn't feel like your situation is working for you or that you are forgotten, that all things are working towards your good. Perhaps, you have a different story and did not receive those types of messages from your mother. Maybe she passed away when you were young or your relationship with your mother was not as nurturing as you would have desired. Whether the type of connect you may have had with your mother was based upon your age at the time of her passing, the kind of relationship that you had, or they type of nurturing connection that you to possessed, you may still feel as though you may have been forgotten due to your experience. As you continue to read through these pages, my hope for you is that you will build upon your faith, discover the purpose for your story, and continue to learn principles that you can use within the context of your life. Let's start with the vision of all things working together for good—your good, and also the good of God's purpose being worked out in your life.

Reason For Courage

It takes courage to face our pain and to take action to heal after a mother has passed away from cancer. It may have been a long journey during the time of her health challenge. As with any major undertaking, we all must start with a vision. A vision is what we see for our future. Our vision feeds into our greater purpose. In the Word of God, it says:

> *"Where there is no vision, the people cast off restraint..."*
> *Proverbs 29:18 (ASV)*

Therefore, begin to cultivate a vision for your life. Visualize your healing, restoration, joy, and happiness.

Our mothers may have been considered the best women we know or irreplaceable. We may always miss her, but that does not equate that we have to remain stuck in despair. I tend to visualize that when a person loses a mother that person who experiences the loss sort of becomes inducted into a sorority or fraternity with similar individuals connected through the common experience of loss and pain. Each person understands the pain of that loss. Therefore, you can create great relationships with others who have had similar situations as a result of this season. When you have lost a mother, and you hear of or notice someone who has experienced that same type of loss, you may find that you can identify with him or her and have compassion about his or her situation.

In times of grief and loss, especially after a long battle against cancer, a person can become more vulnerable to unhealthy relationships. They can let their guard down, and open the doors to unhealthy and toxic relationships to help cope with the pain that they are suffering. This includes friend choices and intimate relationships. Be careful of relationships that are used to escape the realities of life. It takes courage to face the truth and to receive your healing. In some cases, it takes courage to admit to having toxic relationships due to the hurt from loosing a mother, and taking action to break away from them so that you can obtain to fullness of your healing. If you or any person were to choose to keep those unhealthy relationships in their life, it will hinder the progress of grief recovery.

Courage is not just for you, but also for those around you such as your children or the legacy of the person who has passed away. Because cancer affects so many women, they all have a journey and a story of their own. Courage is the hallmark of all of the special women who fight against cancer and other sicknesses. The courage and strength that it takes to stand against a health challenge makes our mothers some of the bravest women we have ever known.

Like many, my mother walked through her journey with courage and joy through breast cancer. My mother wanted to be remembered in a positive light and she accomplished that goal. She lived well. Most mothers want their children and family to remember them in a happy and positive way. As a mother, I too would want my children to remember me as courageous, happy, full of faith, and with unconditional love for them all. I would want my children to live on happy and confident if anything were to ever happen to me no matter how old they were or how old I was at the time. I would want them to be authentic, live purposed, and follow Christ with all of their hearts. Our vision for how we would want others to live is the catalyst to stimulate our healing and growth during a hard time. Do you have someone in your life that if something were to happen to you, that you would want them to live on and move on in a positive way? If so, then embrace that vision and allow for that vision to be a part of your motivation and inspiration to help you travel through the path of grief recovery. Many times, we may come across obstacles in our lives and we cannot see the light at the end of the tunnel for ourselves, but the love we have for someone else gives us clarity on how to make it to the other side of our pain. In the journey of healing, we have to be courageous and positive to live out the destiny that we have been called to live. Therefore, be authentic with your story, intentional about your healing, and pursue your vision for restoration with all of your heart.

Work Unseen

"How can things be working for my good when I feel so bad?" I thought. After my mother passed away, I learned that it's easy to believe in the things that we can see, but it is another thing to believe in what we cannot see. Losing a mother to breast cancer almost seemed unbearable. I thought to myself, how could there be any good in any of this?

I am discovering that not all healing miracles are physical healings.

Even when it seems that there is not anything positive working for us, there is. Some miracles take place in our hearts and minds. We may not see anything working in our favor after our mother passes away, but by faith, we must believe that this too shall pass. The shock and pain of the loss of a mother can cause just as much damage to the soul as physical damage caused in an accident. Wouldn't it then be necessary to seek God to heal our hearts, just as it would be if we needed healing if we were injured in an accident? Therefore, not all healings are physical. The healings of our soul is just as important as the healing of our body. We should approach the healing of our soul with the same confidence and faith as we would if we wanted a physical healing. If your soul feels sad, I encourage you to engage your grief recovery with confidence, faith, and love

We may not always feel like things are working out for us. I want to encourage you to have faith that things are working out in your favor. The road may not be easy, but it will get better. The light at the end of the tunnel will get brighter as you continue to move by faith towards your recovery. One day, you will reflect on this season and see the many great things that you have learned. One day, the promise of things working together for you will resonate and bring joy like never before.

All Things Work Together
Making It Personal

What do you see working together for your good in the future? What could you do to walk in courage in this season of life? What vision do you have for your life? What is your vision for your future? What actions could you take to trust in what is unseen despite what you may be seeing at the moment?

Clarity For The Grieving

"I am still going to continue on my journey of grief and healing. It's hard, and it's painful, but I hope one day that my life will find meaning and purpose again. There have been so many life-changing events at one time. Typically, I can get through things very easily and quickly, but not this. Therefore, there must be a lesson in this for me to travel this path for so long. I know that as a Believer, I should be in a state of peace, wholeness, healing, and restoration, but I don't have that right now. Father, please give me clarity on how to grieve. Show me how to get through this. What is it that you want me to learn? I am tired of people being unreal with me or giving advice that haven't gone through this path. Please help me to get clear and get healed."

~ *Journal Entry*

Grief, Mourning, and Bereavement

You may have questions about your mother's death such as: "How do I move on?" "Will it ever get easier?" "Why did she have to die?" "How do I grieve?" or "How can I have a new normal?" Getting clarity on how to deal with the pain and all of your questions is a key step to your recovery.

Grief affects people in different ways. We must commit ourselves to the healing process no matter how painful or uncertain it may appear along the way. If you want to regain health, reclaim your happiness, and be prosperous in every area of your life, you have to take small steps towards grief recovery. Here are the definitions of grief, mourning, and bereavement:

> ***Grief*** *is the emotional reaction to loss.*
> ***Mourning*** *is the outward expression of grief.*
> ***Bereavement*** *is the state of grief.*

Most people will grieve when they lose a mother, *but not all mourn*. Grief is the emotional reaction to loss. Grief is how we respond to or our initial reaction to our loss.

The pain of loss may require additional support. I needed the support of prayer partners and god-sisters to keep me above water. If it wasn't for my prayer partners and god-sisters I don't know what I would have done at certain times. They were my rock. We prayed, cried, and vented together. They supported me along the way because we genuinely cared for each other. Plus, we found that once one person would go through the situation that another person would experience the same situation. Therefore, the support continued to rotate throughout our circle of sisterhood. What I loved most about my tribe of like-minded and like-faith sisters was that we prayed for each other, allowed for each person to be authentic in their emotions, and gently held each other accountable to leaning towards Christ in a judgment free environment. We shared moments of sadness and hilarious commentaries. I highly recommend getting connected or creating a tribe to help support you through this journey because it will help you to properly express your grief and to mourn.

While grief is what we do internally, mourning is what we do *externally* to express the pain of the loss. For example, mourning is when people dress all in black, cry, or do something externally to express their pain. Therefore, when I say that most people do not mourning, I am saying that they are not outwardly expressing what they are feeling internally. For most people, in order to move forward, they need to mourn. When a person cries or fasts, it allows for their body and spirit to express what is going on inside, and many times that action of mourning is what is necessary to obtain closure and find healing. If you are one of those people who prefers to bottle things up, then you may want to consider thinking about how you can start mourning. Even though you may have cried or expressed pain upon the initial news as a reaction to your mother's passing or at the funeral, you may have never just taken the time to mourn.

When it comes to your healing after losing your mother, please allow me to share some advice to take your time and take the time to heal. Your journey of grief recovery is about knowing your truth, speaking your truth, and living out your truth. Don't rush yourself or allow anyone else to rush you through your process. But do take the actions to do what is necessary to get to the other side of your pain. One of the purposes in this step of the process is to become unstuck, mourn, and not to become stagnant. Therefore, our work in grief recovery is to lean forward towards our healing. You owe it to yourself to be free and to live healthy. Take the time to be healthy and gain your life back.

Slowly but surely, day by day, month-by-month, and year-by-year, you will get stronger and better. The experience of your mother passing is not about making this experience your end but the start of a new beginning in your new normal. This is a start of a new era that includes hope, faith, and total prosperity in your life if you take action and go through your process. Let's think about it for a moment. When a King or Queen dies, the kingdom is not forsaken but passed on to their children. The world needs you to continue and function as the person you were destined to be. This is the start of your new normal in wholeness and with clarity. It reminds me of a comforting scripture that I used during my time of grief:

> "Even though I walk through the darkest valley, I will fear no evil, for you are with me; your rod and your staff, they comfort me."
> Psalm 23:4

There isn't any reason to fear or feel alone because He is always with us.

Grief Is A Process

Most people do not recognize that they have entered into stages of grief immediately after their mother passes away. For example, have you ever seen someone accidentally walk out of the bathroom with a piece of tissue stuck at the bottom of his or her shoe? Have you ever seen someone accidentally walk out of the bathroom with a piece of toilet tissue stuck at the bottom of his or her shoe? The tissue is stuck to the person's shoe, but they are unaware of it. It isn't until someone else brings to their attention about the fact that there is a piece of tissue at the bottom of their shoe that they notice that it's there. Once it is brought to their attention, they immediately jump to remove it. That is what can happen with the grief process. There are times when people are unaware that they have grief and hurt. They are walking around with it, carrying it, and lugging it around. Yet, they are not conscience of this fact. They are stuck in limbo and don't know it. They are stuck in a place in their life or emotions after losing their mother.

Our pain should be addressed through the process of grieving and mourning because the pain of losing a mother can show up elsewhere in our lives. We have to deal with our truth as it relates to our pain if we want to see success in our lives.

Stages Of Grief

The stages of grief are phases that help us frame and identify what we are feeling. You may be able to identify where you are in your journey of grief recovery after looking over this list. Or there may be a person that you care about who is going through the loss of a mother, and this list will help you to better identify where they are in the journey based upon some of the behaviors that you may have seen. The five stages of grief are:

1. Shock and Denial
2. Anger
3. Bargaining
4. Depression
5. Acceptance and Hope

There is not a timetable as to how long a person will take in each stage. A person could have a combination of these feelings during their grief process or fail to reach the Acceptance stage of their journey, for example. So let's look at the symptoms that we can notice about our behavior and life when we lose a mother that may help us to identify where we are in the stages of grief. Here is a list of some of the most common symptoms:

- Anxiety, panic, and fear
- Disorganization, confusion, searching, and yearning
- Explosive emotions
- Physiological changes (including difficulties with eating and sleeping, as well as diminished energy)
- Guilt, remorse, and assigning blame
- Feelings of loss, emptiness, and sadness
- Feelings of relief and release.

We owe it to ourselves to take care of our health and well-being. Identify where you are in the process and take courage to move forward through the stages of grief. In my case, it was losing my mother to an illness and how to deal with it.

Myths About Grief

There are many myths about what grief is and how to deal with it. These myths appear in our everyday lives such as at home, work, and church and create confusion. By being real in our journey of grief recovery, not only do we obtain the freedom and healing that we desire, but helps point others to Christ, who is the real Superhero in our lives during the process. It also shows people that in the midst of our storms, our sin, our imperfections, our flaws, that Christ still loved us enough to be patient and long-suffering to deliver us out of our pain.

Here are eight common myths about grief. Perhaps you have heard of or seen some of them yourself during the course of your journey. Let's go through each one of them:

Myth #1:	God does not want us to grieve
Myth #2:	God will get angry with us if we grieve
Myth #3:	We should only be happy
Myth #4:	We should not cry or mourn
Myth #5:	My emotions are a sign of weak faith
Myth #6:	My grief means that I do not trust God
Myth #7:	My faith has failed
Myth #8:	My prayers did not work

These myths are not only false but can be damaging to a person's relationship with God. These myths can confuse someone into believing that God is out to hurt them or to cause them harm. Pastors, churches, non-profits, and the community should inquire about and consider having resources, small groups, and programs in their church to address the well-balanced truth of God's word when it comes to grief after a losing a mother to cancer. In my case, it was losing a mother to cancer and how to deal with it.

Our souls can be renewed, refreshed, and restored! When we take time each day to identify the goodness that is around us we can renew ourselves and travel through the grief process. If you have noticed any of these myths in your life or someone else's, make the decision to remove these myths from your life and to start living in truth.

Permission To Not Be Okay

Give yourself permission to not be okay in order to get to a place that is acceptable. Allow yourself for the moment to be the person who lost their mother and not a superman or superwoman who has everything under control. Try your best to avoid wearing the mask and putting on an act to appease and appeal to everyone else. Let's be clear about whom this truth also pertains to. This truth pertains to those who are in the church as well. Church members or believers can wear a mask and act as if everything is all right. Even as a believer, it is acceptable for you to not be yourself and to have some concerns in your life! You must be real with yourself and your feelings if you are to step into your healing and begin to walk in a journey that will help you to overcome the loss of your parent.

Grief, Mourning, and Bereavement
Making It Personal

What does it mean to grieve, mourn, or be in bereavement? What areas of your life would you like to see healed from being broken? Did you recognize any of the grief symptoms? If so, which ones? Did you recognize any of the myths about grief? If so, which ones? How have they affected your healing process?

"My heart aches for my mother and I know I need to move forward, but I don't know where to start. Some days I feel sad and others I feel like everything will be okay. All I know is that I want to get through this but I don't know what steps to take. I'm getting so much advice but it isn't always real or relatable to my life. Father, guide me through this path with faith so that I may gain better understanding."

~ Journal Entry

How Do I Grieve Or Mourn?

The journey of grief is unique for each person. It is important to know that the steps set out below are just guidelines, like the bumpers down a bowling alley. This is not a comprehensive list. Recovery is a process, and it is different for each person. The reason why it is different is because each person and relationship is different.

Some people may have had a great relationship with their mother, while others may not have. Some people may have lost their mother when they were very young and did not have the opportunity to get to spend as much time with her or know her as much. Or they may not have had the opportunity to grieve at a younger age and now want to take the steps to freedom from that grief. The list can go on and on.

In order to successfully grieve and come to a place of solace, you must come to terms with the loss, learn how to cope, and move forward into your new normal.

Here are seven steps that I took during my own recovery and that you can take to start your own grief recovery process if you choose: you can

1. **Be Intentional About Your Healing**

    Decide to have faith and be intentional throughout your recovery. Facing your fears and taking on grief recovery requires faith and courage. The death of a loved one can be a painful experience for those who are left behind. Take actions daily such as daily affirmation, positive thinking, and doing something that you enjoy.

For some, getting to the other side of grief will take intentional actions. You can discover wholeness and freedom by being intentional about your healing.

2. **Lean Forward Into Your Healing**

   Next, you want to do what I call leaning forward into your healing. This means that you are actively taking steps towards the direction of your healing. You aren't simply waiting for recovery to jump into your lap, but you are taking action to facilitate that healing. You could do this by reading, relaxing, exercising, cooking, or starting a new hobby that will positively reinforce your healing.

3. **Weeping Is Good For The Soul**

   Remember the passage of scripture:

   > *"...weeping may stay for the night, but rejoicing comes in the morning."*
   > *Psalm 30:5*

   Weeping or crying is good for the soul. When we weep it helps us to heal. Sometimes we need to have a good cry, or what some call the "ugly cry." Crying is not weak or cowardly. It is a sign of strength and courage to allow the tears to flow from your eyes in a way that allows you to heal, to move forward, and to be empowered. Weeping releases the emotions that we have buried. You may need to find a place to go to be alone to let it all hang out. Wherever that may be for you, be sure to allow yourself some time to weep.

4. **Take The Time And Take Your Time**

   There is not a timetable for grief recovery because it affects each of us differently. Our goal is to go through the process in as healthy a way as possible and to heal and move forward. You do not want to use this part as an excuse to stay stuck or to maintain unresolved issues. This is the place to be authentically okay and to receive your healing.

5. **Share Your Truth**

    Don't be afraid to communicate where you are in your journey with your loved ones. If you are hurting or struggling, be honest with them. If the passing is affecting your mood, attitudes and decisions, be sure to communicate to them about how you are feeling. Be sure to take positive actions to address the mood swings and attitudes because it can negatively affect the relationships around you.

6. **Find Scriptures That Will Comfort And Strengthen You**

    Get scriptures that will encourage and comfort you. Place them on an index card, your phone, journal, or any place that is easily accessible. Be sure to find words that will encourage you in your faith and in your daily life. Find the scriptures that deal with your specific issue or concern. Find stories in the Bible about people who have had the same experience. In the back of this book, there is a list of a few scriptures for comfort and strength. Find the ones that resonate with you, and create your confessions to help you in your healing.

7. **Encourage Yourself In The Lord**

    Be sure to encourage yourself in the Lord daily. Encourage yourself with worship, praise, and thinking of positive things that make you happy or bring joy to you. This part of the journey can also tie into #6, by which you will encourage yourself in the Lord as you say your confessions. During my journey, I would stand up, look into the mirror, and make my confessions or affirmations every day. I wrote in my journal daily. Decide what actions you will take daily to be encouraged.

Remember, when we take steps towards grief recovery we are nursing ourselves back to health.

Grief recovery is about recovering from a loss to get to place of normality. Just because you are in recovery doesn't mean you do not mourn or have pain, it means that you are taking the right steps and medicine to get back to a place of wholeness. Our medicine during this time is the Word of God, faith, and hope. You may still have your moments of brief sadness triggered by a song on the radio, a favorite television show, or a common hobby, and that is okay. That is the time when we cry our tears and then take our medicine. By faith, it will get better. Day by day, we will receive the promise of healing.

Letting Go

When the reality set in that my mother had passed away, in my eyes the thought of being without her was far worse than dealing with the pain of letting her go. If I were honest with myself, I did not want to let go because I did not want to let go of my pain. I felt as though I was betraying her if I accepted her death and moved on with my life. For me, the mere thought of acknowledging that she had passed away was more painful than the reality of living without her. I did not look forward to the future because I was uncertain of what would come up or could happen.

I was really close to my mother. Not only did I have to come to terms with the idea that I had lost my mother, but I also had to come to terms with the idea that I no longer had the position of being a daughter to a mother. Deep down inside, I knew that I would have to let go if I were to move forward. By this time, I had a little girl and another one on the way. I felt as though my children did not deserve to have a mother who was not whole and complete. So, I made the decision to continue in faith to claim my healing and to start the journey of letting go.

Letting go is a lot easier said than done. But so many times, we can find ourselves stuck in a place of not letting go or being in limbo. Making the decision to take the step towards letting go is crucial in the healing process. There is healing and restoration on the other side. We can recover from loss by letting go.

Recovery will take time. It will take time to get to the point where you can function without that loved one in your life. It may take some time to gain closure. You are the one who decides how you will take this journey. Giving yourself time to grieve and heal allows you to properly process how to get back to or discover a place of normality. Learning how to grieve and mourn the loss of our mother is one of the most important steps. If you need additional help with this process, I highly encourage you to seek a well-balanced grief counselor. Doing so can be refreshing and helpful if needed in this process.

Give yourself permission to mourn. Allow yourself that time to open up about your feelings and what you are going through. You will make it. You will discover how to experience joy again and how to live your life with purpose and happiness again. Decide today to surrender to the possibilities of what good things can take place in your life.

How Do I Grieve Or Mourn?
Making It Personal

What do you know now about how to mourn that you did not know before? What actions can you start taking to express mourning about your mother to assist with the healing process? In the back of the book, there are scriptures on healing and comfort; which scriptures can you begin to meditate on and confess?

Big Boys...And Men...Do Cry

> *"Believe me, every heart has its secret sorrows, which the world knows not, and oftentimes we call a man cold, when he is only sad."*
> ~ Henry Wadsworth Longfellow: Hyperion, Book III Chapter IV

Big Boys...And Men...Do Cry

"Boys don't cry!" "Be a man!" "Don't be a wimp!" is what most boys will hear as they grow up. Our society tends to teach boys from a young age that showing emotion is a sign of weakness. This type of behavior is taught to and learned by young boys everywhere and carried over as the norm into male adulthood. The issue with this philosophy is that boys and men are human beings with real emotional connections just as women are. If a man is not allowed to be himself, he can begin to feel undervalued or underappreciated by those who are around him because he did not get to properly deal with his pain.

There can be differences in the ways that men and women express the pain of losing a mother. A woman may easily cry all of the time and talk about her pain with many people. Some men, however, may not choose to express their pain with their words in the same way. Both men and women deal with grief in their own way and should be allowed to do so. Losing a mother can be hard on anyone. It is important to give grace to people as they go through that journey.

Most people tend to lend helping hands and support to women who have experienced the loss of a mother, but what do we do about our men and our boys who have lost their mothers? Who is thinking about the son, father, or husband who just lost their mother to an illness?

Men and boys can have some of the deepest levels of love and appreciation for their mothers. Their hearts break and grieve just as much as women's. Behind the scenes, our boys and men are hurting. They could fall short of reaching their best potential if they do not embrace the truth about their pain. One of the best ways that a boy or man can honor the legacy and memory of their mother is by allowing them to open up about their pain and heal from their loss by seeking God. There is a good example of a strong man in the Lord, named David, who sought God in the time of despair in the book of Psalms:

> *"Hear my cry, O God; listen to my prayer. From the ends of the earth I call to you, I call as my heart grows faint; lead me to the rock that is higher than I. For you have been my refuge, a strong tower against the foe. I long to dwell in your tent forever and take refuge in the shelter of your wings."*
> *Psalm 61:1-4*

In the book of Psalms, David is praying in a time of despair. He is crying unto the Lord because his heart is faint. David is praying to God his midst of distress. He shares his desire to be rescued by God from his pain. David lays aside his ego and opens up to God in prayer in a manner that any man can do. Sure, David had his flaws, but even with his flaws David was considered a man after God's own heart in Acts 13:22.

Perhaps you or someone you know believes that they are unworthy of being able to approach God in prayer because they don't feel that they are connected to God, made mistakes in the past, or are turned off by religion. Receiving your healing from God does not require that you attend a church building or be a perfect individual. You can receive your healing in a hotel room, office building, in your car, or wherever you feel that you are in a safe place to seek God for His help.

Our mothers are our first teachers and irreplaceable. Don't be the person who tries to be Mr. Macho while allowing hurt and pain to cause dysfunction in your relationships, career, and business. When we are on the subject of mother or "momma," there is no such thing as softness, weaknesses, or being wimps because we are mourning the loss of an Irreplaceable Mother! Great athletes, world leaders, and famous scientists have all thanked and loved their mothers. It is okay to be a momma's boy whether you were one in her life or not. It may be necessary to mourn the relationship that you *desired* or *wished* you could have. This is your time to take off all of your titles, responsibilities, and egos—and just be your mother's son.

If the boy is young, then attempt to get him into an environment where he can express his pain in a healthy way. You may notice that he has expressions of his emotions. Perhaps you notice anger, sadness, or temper tantrums. These are indicators that he may not know how to express his hurt about how much he love and miss his mother in a healthy way. Remember, the idea of being a tough guy starts at a young age for some boys. Therefore, allowing for a young child to see vulnerability, express their vulnerability, and know that it is okay to miss their mother may be helpful in their healing process. Overall, it may be best to allow that child to engage in the process of grief recovery and their feelings at an early age so that they can have productive and healthy relationships in the future when they are adults.

If any of this resonates with you, pray and ask for help to become vulnerable and open to change and transformation. Transformation means to change in form, thinking, behavior, appearance, nature, or character. We all must have the freedom to grieve and mourn in a healthy way without condemnation, fear, or judgment. Ask the Lord to soften your heart and give you the strength to pray like David did. Decide today to pray in the seasons of despair with hope—hope of brighter days and deliverance.

Remember, you can do this. You can mourn and move forward after the passing of an Irreplaceable Mother no matter what condition or state you may be in today. Healing is not reserved only for women but for anyone and everyone who wants to be healed, whole, and free in their new normal.

Big Boys…And Men…Do Cry
Making It Personal

What has society told you about how boys and men should respond to pain? What is the most important priority for you to achieve by grieving the passing of your mother? What other issues are important to you? What would you like to see improved? What are some of the best things that you have learned by discovering the meaning of transformation and deliverance in your grief recovery process?

Overcoming Despair

"The passing of my mother was the most painful and memorable time of my life thus far...I still haven't grasped the loss of my mother because it seems like so many things have fallen apart after she left. Every morning, as I get my child ready for daycare, she's full of joy. She's smiling, laughing, and wants me to give her a big hug and a kiss. In that moment, I have so much joy and happiness. In that same moment, I get sad and angry because I have to figure out how to be her mother without a mother... It still seems unreal, as if I will wake up from this bad nightmare. Yet, I push through the pain to try to my best to be the best mother—a happy and whole mother, but it's hard. I know I can do this. There have been many who have travelled this road before me and I know that He is no respecter of persons. I don't see how I will make it, but I know that I will. Lord, help me get out this ditch. I don't see it today, but I hope to escape this despair."

~ Journal Entry

Is This A Bad Nightmare?

In the darkest moments of our lives, there is still hope. The dark cloud of despair may appear so thick over our lives during the times of loss that we are barely able to see what is in front of us. I have learned in my journey that the road of grief and despair isn't covered by a dark fog, but is guided by a beam of light like a lighthouse in the midst of the sea; that light is the love of God. In the beginning, grief appears to be the worst thing that you could imagine, but by the grace of God, the fog will begin to fade, and you will begin to see the light. This is what often happens with our grief and recovery. During my grief, the love of my daughter helped save me. In my journal entry, I had conflicting emotions. I was overjoyed with being a mother. Yet, I struggled on the inside with my pain. The love for my daughter was the love and light that eventually pulled me towards my healing, even though I was having a hard time.

After my mother passed of breast cancer, as I mentioned, I lost my way, my purpose, and vision. However, in the midst of major loss, pain, or setback I was being set up for major redesign and reconstruction. In the same way, you may feel that you have lost your way, purpose, and vision. Yet, in this particular season, our way of life and thinking must now be rebuilt. For example, when a major highway is under construction, especially in a major city, it seems as though the construction will last forever. It could take months or even years to complete a new road, depending on what is being developed. Our journey of recovery involves redesigning our life and then reconstructing it according to the new design, piece by piece, and it can take time. You may have been in a panic, feeling hopeless; but you are not hopeless, because there is hope for you to overcome this situation and season in your life.

The Moment Of Truth

My mother received her treatment at a major cancer center in downtown Detroit. One of the last times that I was able to hang out with her was right after she had a surgery. I went to visit her at the hospital and check on her condition. When I arrived, she was sitting in her room, eating, and talking with a nurse. I sat down to spend time with her and enjoyed that moment because we hung out by ourselves. Most of the time there was someone else there. So, I valued the one on one time.

My mother was having a hard time speaking. Even though she was in the hospital and could barely speak, she managed to get out a smile or short humorous sentences. We decided to watch television because my mom loved TV. The television options were limited, and we were trying to find something we could enjoy. I scrolled to a channel with the Oprah Winfrey show, and she began to smile and point to the TV, saying, "Yes!" I said, "Oprah it is!" and we both laughed.

My mother was always a big Oprah fan. She referred to Oprah as "My Oprah." There's much speculation about and study of the so-called "Oprah effect." I can say that if any of those studies took into account people who were like my mother, then Oprah's influence was definitely top notch in our family. My mom loved anything that Oprah loved, and hated anything that Oprah hated. My mother always admired her and her love for people. My mother had her own list of favorite entertainers. She would always talk well of Oprah to all of us, and the R&B legend Luther Vandross, but that is a story for another day. My mother and I sat together at the hospital, and we had a great time watching the Oprah Winfrey show. Looking back, as I was visiting in the hospital room, I was still in denial. I still did not want to believe what was going on. I could not allow my mind to go down that path to think about it.

The next day, I attended another doctor's appointment. The doctor stated that things weren't looking too good for my mom, but they were still working with her and were planning to give her more medication. They did not mention anything about the fact that she was on the brink of passing away. I left the hospital to get to work. I pulled into the parking lot of my office building at work and received a phone call stating that my mother was being placed in hospice. I was shocked! The doctor did not mention hospice care when I was at the hospital a few moments earlier. I was so shaken that I sat in the parking lot where I worked and cried. I called my manager at the office and said that I was unable to come in. I literally could not walk into the building because I felt that I may have collapsed in the lobby elevator or cried in the middle of a meeting. I could not move my legs to get from the car to the building. I wasn't in a state of mind to face anyone because I simply could not pull it together. I kept saying to myself, *"Get it together, Rin. Shake it off, Rin."* I was known by three main nicknames Rin, Ri, or Lorin. Most of my childhood friends called me Rin. I was envisioning myself surrounded by all of my sister-friends and brothers encouraging me and trying to shake off the negative feelings. But I could not. I finally ended up driving off the lot and went to the house to help prepare for my mother to go home for the hospice.

When my mother arrived at her home, she appeared fine. She was smiling and laughing. She kept her composure and remained in good spirits. I called and insisted that all of my sisters and my youngest brother come over to the house to speak with our mom to say their final words. I was still operating in "big sister mode." I wanted to make sure that each of my siblings had the opportunity to speak with our mother to say their last goodbyes to her before she went home to be with the Lord. Our mother's mom, our grandmother, whom we lovingly call Granny, and my mother's sister, our aunt, were staying with my mother to help take care of her and the house.

After everyone spoke his or her last words, I was able to take a small break. Even though I was in a protective caregiver mode, ensuring that each person spoke with her, I still did not accept that she would pass away soon. My siblings assumed their own natural roles as well. Later that evening, I began to prepare to leave my mother's house to go home for the night to get some rest, as I was leaving my mother's room I turned around and said, "I love you, mommy. See you in the morning!" She said, "Okay sweetie, I love you too, mommy's baby. See you in the morning!" I left the house and drove home. I did not realize that that was going to be the last time that I would speak to my mother or see her alive.

Early the next morning, my father called me and gave me the news that my mother had passed away. I was numb when he told me the news. I woke my husband up and got our daughter dressed to go to my mother's house. When I entered the house, I walked into the room where she laid and began to shake her wrist. I attempted to pick up her arm but her arm was heavy. In a small, feeble voice, I whispered, *"Mommy?"* and she did not answer. I shook her wrist again, only a little harder, and said, *"Mommy?"* She did not answer. My mother was gone. I thought that we had at least a few more days or weeks, but we only had hours.

My mother was a beautiful, brown-skinned Trinidadian woman. She was an immigrant from Trinidad and Tobago who later became an American citizen. As she laid in rest in her bed, her face had a bright shine as though a light came across her body. Her skin looked as though there was a layer of sunshine underneath. She looked peaceful, as though she had just fallen asleep. Her body was still warm, but she was gone home to be with the Lord. I remember every breath I took in that moment. It was as if I had to intentionally force myself to breathe.

I did not know it at the time, but in that moment, in the very second that I realized that my mother had passed away, my soul became *stuck*. My body moved on, and I physically went about the day, but in the moment that she passed away, there was a part of me that died also. My inner soul became frozen in time. In that moment, I was lost. I did not know what to do. I did not realize that I had become stuck until over a year later. I was the person who had everything under control and 'knew it all'. Yet, for the first time in my life, I did not have anything under control and was unclear about my next steps.

The whole thing seemed like a nightmare that did not want to end. I was totally unclear about how I was going to make it. I felt like it was a Freddy Krueger movie or something. I was not at peace. I was just numb. I was just surviving. I was waiting to wake up from my slumber.

In the same way, you may be able to relate to this type of soul slumber, as though this season of your life is a bad nightmare. Be encouraged, that you are not alone in how you feel or your experiences. Our initial response varies from person to person, and there is not a right or wrong way to react to a trauma or life-changing event. There are many others who can resonate with the story and pain of being stuck. This is the place in our journey where we can begin to identify when and where, if applicable, we became stuck. I became stuck when I realized that she passed away. When was the moment for you?

Come on Mom, Pick Up!

Even though my mother had passed away a few weeks earlier, it did not really sink in. I was on autopilot and did not realize that I was stuck yet. I went about my life business as usual. My husband and I were planning to close on our new home. The final updates and repairs to the house were made, and all of the inspections were completed. We were finally in the position to get the keys. I woke up early on the day of our closing. After the closing, my husband and I felt great! We were homeowners again! I rushed to our new home to soak in the moment.

My husband and I hugged and kissed as we basked in homeownership, for this was the house that we were going to grow our family. I hurried to grab my cell phone to call my mother to tell her about the closing. I was excited about telling her the news and hearing her voice. The phone rang and rang. I thought to myself, *"Come on mom, and pick up!"* I hung up and called her again. Once again, the phone continued ringing, and she did not answer. I started to get irritated, wondering where she was and why she hadn't picked up. On the third call, it finally hit me! *"Oh wait! She is not there! She had passed away."* Shaking my head in almost disbelief, staring at my phone, my mother's voicemail came on again. In that moment, I realized for the first time in weeks, that my mother had really passed away. I stood in one spot completely frozen. It was as if I were having an out-of-body experience. I looked down at my hands to see if they were really there. I could not take it in. I helped plan the funeral and attended the funeral. But the reality of the event had not set in.

Shock is a sudden upsetting or surprising event or experience.

Could it have been that I was in shock and/or denial? Or was that I was "choosing" not to believe that she has passed away? Shock and denial have many layers. Perhaps you are like how I was, a person who did not want to believe the new reality or were on autopilot. I thought to myself, *what if I didn't want a new life or new normal? What if the pain of feeling stuck in all of my anguish and hurt was less painful than the truth of my reality?* The fear of the unknown seemed less painful than accepting that my mother had passed away. Trying to live on without my mother, my best friend felt like it would be a betrayal. Denial? Yes, I was in denial. Shock? Yes, I was in shock. And I wasn't sure if I wanted to move forward out of that stage of my grief.

When a mother passes away of an illness, and in my case my mother passed of cancer, we may experience the emotions of shock and denial. It does not matter how long of a process, how many chemo appointments we attended, or how many organic smoothies we created. If our loved one passes away, it could feel like a sudden upset to our lives. Their passing could have caused an interruption in the routine of our lives, and you could find yourself feeling as though you are floating through life. This reminds me of when the astronaut, Neil Armstrong, walked the moon for the first time; he floated for a few seconds between each step as he walked across the moon. During this journey, we could feel as though we are floating through time and space from one place to the next. That may be due to the fact that we are in shock or denial.

Sweet Dreams

The good news is that when a person loses their mother, they are not floating through time and space without any love or assistance. Though it may feel like we are going through life aimlessly, there is an amazing purpose and plan for our lives working in the background. God has not forgotten or forsaken us. He is aware and understands all of our emotions, lifestyles, and questions. Therefore, we can experience rest and sweet dreams because He is right there ready to comfort, heal, and restore.

Is This A Bad Nightmare?
Making It Personal

What would being in shock or denial look like in your situation? What was your moment of truth? How did you process your moment of truth? How do you feel about the passing of your mother and are you in a place where her passing has become a 'reality' in your life? What positive things do you think you could begin to do to start the journey of accepting her passing, in order to move toward your healing and new normal?

"This is not real. You have to be kidding me. This is a lot of mess. I just wish sometimes that the Lord would come back right now and take us all up! Save me the journey of having to suffer in this life and face the fact that my mom is not here. Save me headache of having to hear people tell me that this is not a big deal. Who are they to judge me? I can't even lose my mother without people expecting perfection from me. At times, I just want to scream or go off on people for the things they say and do. I know my attitude is bad right now and I need to fix it. But I am just confused and hurt. I don't accept this as my life. Father, help me understand this season and keep my faith."
~ Journal Entry

I Don't Accept This!

Like many, I found myself making excuses about my current condition. I denied my reality and truth even though they were staring me right in the face. I said, *"No, this can't be happening to me."* My life was changing and headed towards an unknown path. My life, family dynamic, and traditions were shifting but this time without a matriarch at the head of it. Bringing myself to a place to admit that my mother had passed away from cancer was difficult. Deep down inside I knew that I needed to face my truth and stop floating through life if I were to ever get healed of my pain. I had to admit that my life had changed, that my mother has passed away, and that it was okay; and that I would be okay.

In order to understand denial, we must discuss the definition of denial. I found this definition:

Denial is failing to admit that something has occurred when it has or the action of declaring something to be untrue.

Denying our reality does not make it any more or less of a reality. However, denying our reality could hinder us from reaching our highest potential and healing, because when we are in denial about our situation, we are also denying our truth.

Transformation takes place in the company of truth.

Transformation is possible when we face our realities, rather than denying them. This may not happen overnight. However, accepting the fact that this part of the process must take place is a step towards recovery and healing.

Feeling Numb

I felt numb for a long time after my mother passed away. Numbness is also a normal reaction to a death or loss. However, be careful not to confuse numbness with not caring. Being numb means to be disconnected emotionally from the situation. People tend to do this as a way to protect them from feeling additional pain. In doing so, it could cause further feelings of hopelessness and despair.

A good example of what being numb would look like is my experience of the winter season when our family lived in Michigan. The first snow at the beginning of winter was always fun. My friends and I would go out to play, making snowmen, and having snow fights. After playing in the snow for hours, all of us would run into the house because we were freezing cold. I would cry out to my parents, "I can't feel my fingers or my toes!" The pain that was in my hands and feet was almost unbearable. Therefore, taking into consideration this example, one side of this scenario was that I was numb. I couldn't feel anything. Yet, at the same time, I was in pain that was almost unbearable. In the same way, when our mother passes away, we could feel numb and have pain at the same time.

Confronting our truth and acknowledging it if we are numb and in pain will aid in the recovery process. Numbness does not mean the absence of pain. Pain does not mean the absence of numbness. It is possible to have both. One way that I confronted this issue of numbness was when I went back to work after the funeral. Going back to work was hard. I was numb and had difficulty concentrating. Activities such as attending meetings, writing emails, and having basic conversations had suddenly become very difficult. It was hard to stay focused.

My strategy was to gather a list of scriptures and positive affirmations, and write them and place them in the back of my planner so that I could turn to them throughout the day discreetly to stay encouraged. There were times when I was in a meeting or talking with my fellow peers, and would begin to feel sad about my mother. The emotion would just come to me from out of the blue. I would flip casually to the back of the planner to read a scripture or positive affirmation. I immediately began to feel better. No one in the meeting could tell or knew what I was doing because it was my planner, which was the same place that I kept my meeting notes. I encourage you to take this technique and use it to encourage yourself. Find ways to encourage yourself throughout the day while you are at work, school, or on the go. This will help you to overcome the numbness and denial, and will also encourage you throughout the day.

In your journey, you may deal with feeling as though you are numb while dealing with a lot of pain. It may hurt in your process, but don't quit; there is healing, recovery, and deliverance on the other side. Just as we can get relief from the cold weather by running into a warm house, we can get relief from coldness of grief by running to the warmth and love of God on a daily basis.

The Holy Spirit As The Shock Defender

Despite all that we may go through, we are not left alone. We are blessed with the gift of the Holy Spirit to help us through our times of grief. The Holy Spirit helps minimize the blows of grief and gives comfort during the time of loss. This does not mean that we will not feel anything, but it does mean that we are not alone and that we can take comfort in His love. The Holy Spirit is our guide, our teacher, and Comforter in the times that we need it most. Therefore, allow the Holy Spirit into your journey as your shock defender. He will defend you, protect you, and comfort you.

I Don't Accept This!
Making It Personal

What does feeling numb look like in your world? After reading this section, what things have happened that would have caused you pain, but you were unable to feel it? What affirmations or daily actions could you take to encourage yourself throughout the day? Now that we know that the Holy Spirit is the Shock Defender, how would you like for the Holy Spirit to help and comfort you?

"I must learn to move forward to live a healthy, healed, and happy life. I must move forward so that my children can have joy and an example of how to navigate through life. I don't need to be disingenuous with them, hide my struggles, or flaws. I need to be real, so that they can be real. Truth is, I'm stuck and need to get unstuck. They don't deserve the backlash of any adult drama. I have to get back on course for me and for them. So, what is my purpose now? What I am supposed to do with my life going forward? Father, please, help me. I'm stuck..."

~ Journal Entry

Are You Stuck In Despair?

When an essential person like a mother figure goes home to be with the Lord, it takes some of us off course. Our soul, which is defined generally biblically as "the mind, will, and emotions of a person," tends to veer off course like a ship that has lost its path during its voyage. It is possible to lose sight of our purpose and direction, leaving us with a deep sense of loss as we scramble to rediscover our plan.

My life could have been compared to a person trying hold on to a bar of wet soap. I was trying to get a grip on life, but it was slipping through my hands. I was trying to figure out the meaning of life and how to manage my roles as a wife, a mother, an employee, a family member, and investor. The motivation behind my accomplishments was rooted in pleasing others and my parents, which I discovered was not healthy for me. I was struggling with making connections with God, my husband, my church, my friends, my family—everyone. I found myself getting hurt and angry with others. My attitude was not the best. As I mentioned, the moment I recognized that my mom had passed away, when I called her name but she didn't answer me, I became stuck. The clock on the wall continued to move, but the inner clock of my soul paused.

As the oldest daughter, I spoke at the funeral. I don't know how I was able to get through that and speak on behalf of the family. Our family decided to wear all-white suits or dresses, and have all-white flowers, to symbolize her pure spirit and to have an uplifting ceremony. We did not want to have a sad funeral. We wanted our mother's funeral to be a celebration of her life. Everything came together so nicely, but behind the smiles, there was a pain. I thought that I was strong. I thought I had all of the answers about grief and God. When asked about my mother's passing, I gave all of the perfect Christian responses. Underneath the exterior though, for the first time in my life as a believer, woman, wife, and mother, I was unsure of who I was and my purpose. I was existing, but not living.

We don't always recognize the moment that we became stuck or the fact that it happened. Losing a mother can cause us to lose balance. Fortunately for me, I was able to recognize it during a time of personal prayer and worship.

Avoiding Is Not The Answer

Avoiding the pain is not the answer either. We can't live a healthy life avoiding what happened to us. At some point, we will have to confront the pain, understand what it is, and deal with it.

There are three ways that people try to avoid the pain of loss when it comes to the passing of their mother:

1. **Becoming Busy**

    One way to avoid pain is to become busy with work, extra-curricular activities, family, new projects, and more. It is a way to keep our minds off thinking about the pain of our loss and the fact that our parent is no longer with us. Becoming busy helps distracts us from facing the fact of our reality and thus can hinder our transformation.

2. **Avoiding Places**

    Another way to avoid our reality is to avoid places that you used to go or enjoy with your mother. This would include church, events, networking or social clubs, and even her burial site. The reasoning behind this could be that those places remind us of the deceased and cause sadness. If this is you, become open to allowing for those familiar places to become a place of remembrance and healing.

3. **Portraying An Image**

   Acting as though everything is okay is another way for a grieving person to wear the mask and avoid the issue. On the outside, they could be laughing and smiling, but on the inside, they are very broken and hurt. They portray an image that nothing is wrong. This creates an illusion of perfection that allows for them to avoid the pain of loss.

Grace To Become Unstuck

> *"'My grace is sufficient for you, for my power is made perfect in weakness.'"*
> *2 Corinthians 12:9*

Are you just going through life, living on autopilot or stuck in the midst of your grief recovery after loosing your mother?

A good example of being stuck is when a woman is running down the street in heels to catch up with a friend or a cab, and as she is running the heel of her shoe gets stuck in a crack. She is unable to move forward until she pulls her shoe out of the crack. She may have to yank and pull it before it becomes loose so that she can continue on her journey. In the same way, you may have been headed in a certain direction, and you got stuck. Now, you have to pull yourself out of the cracks to move forward with your journey and new normal.

We are all different people with various backgrounds. It does not matter if you are a man, woman, or child. We all had our own unique relationship with our mothers. No matter what kind of relationship you may have had with your mother, there is grace for your journey, healing, and rebuilding into your new normal after she has passed away. Change is uncomfortable most of the time, but it will produce the greatest reward in our lives if we act upon God's word. God's grace is sufficient and able to sustain us through difficult times. That is the promise and the good news for us all.

Take Off The Mask With Joy

As you take off the mask and get unstuck, you may find it difficult to find your joy. To combat the harsh effects of depression, we must fill ourselves with joy and praise. We can do this by taking time in the Word of God, worship, support groups, counseling, or praise. One familiar passage of scripture is:

> *"Rejoice in the Lord always. I will say it again: Rejoice!"*
> *Philippians 4:4*

During my own journey, I struggled with depression after my mother passed away. It was hard to admit, but I was very sad at the loss. However, I made the decision to focus on more positive things to get to the other side by finding my joy and getting my happy back! By taking the time to rejoice, even when we don't feel like it, we fight against depression and take the focus away from negative things. Depression can be defeated and joy can be received, through rejoicing. Depression does not have to rule over anyone's life once they lose a mother. Making the decision to break free from depression is the best choice a person can make towards their healing. Therefore, make the decision to rejoice on the good things in your life during this season.

Destroying Depression

―•∞•―

"I am pain-stricken. My heart is full of sadness. It isn't getting any better. It feels worse. I haven't talked to her in months. I barely went four days without talking to her. I miss her laugh, her voice, her crazy sayings...I wish my mom was still alive.
But I will praise him anyway. I don't always feel like it, but when I do, I feel peace. Every day I look forward to getter better. Father, please don't leave me here in this sadness. I need to get out."
~ Journal Entry

Destroying Depression With Faith And Prayer

As I have already mentioned, I struggled with depression for a season. I did not realize that I was depressed because I did not have what I believed to be the normal symptoms, such as crying or sleeping all of the time. However, I had other symptoms that identified that I was struggling. I stopped celebrating holidays such as Mother's Day and doing some of the things that my mother and I liked to do. I would go to my mother's burial site, but that was all. She was the reason for giving gifts during those times, and since she was no longer here, I did not feel the need to celebrate them any longer.

Depression is an intense condition that affects millions of people, Christians and non-Christians alike. People who suffer from it experience intense feelings of sadness, hopelessness, fatigue, and anger. Stress caused by the loss of a loved one, a difficult relationship, or traumatic situation can trigger depression. Loosing a mother to cancer qualifies for being an event that can trigger depression in a person's life.

If we aren't careful, depression can hold us hostage. It almost did in my case. I was bound to negative thoughts and the loss of a sense of purpose and passion. I was confused as to how to move forward. The spirit of depression speaks negativity to our inner soul about how we cannot move on. Depression is not our friend. Keep in mind, it is perfectly normal to feel sad when we lose our mother, but it becomes an issue when it begins to affect our desire to live our best lives.

This is what happened to me. I am pretty upbeat, but in this case, I was "heart poor." If my spirit were a car, I would be on "E." If it were not for my daughter, I may not have been able to pull through. At the time I did not love myself enough. I loved my husband, but I viewed him as being an adult and having the ability to be independent. However, when I gazed at my daughters, I decided that I could not allow myself to continue in my current state. I felt as though they did not deserve to have a sad mom but deserved to have a mother who was happy and who loved life. I prayed and asked God to help me.

In the same manner, if you find yourself in depression, ask God to help you to overcome depression so that you can be a happy and healthy person in your life.

Effects Of Depression After Losing A Mother

Depression can occur in more instances than just after loosing a mother. Our focus in this book is on the passing of mothers after a battle with cancer, but as we discuss depression, it can be used for all forms of issues. Many people try keep their feelings bottled up, but their depression may be displayed elsewhere in their life such as in mood swings, poor work performance, drug abuse, alcoholism, low sexual interest or sexual promiscuity, and a lack of self-value and self-worth. Nonetheless, when we are in times of despair, we are not alone even though it may feel like it. There may be times when we feel as though God is far away, but He is not. He is always close. This is proven in this passage of scripture from the book of Psalms:

> *"The Lord is close to the brokenhearted and saves those who are crushed in spirit."*
> *Psalm 34:18*

If a person is experiencing depression and has not processed their grief, it can affect various areas of their life. Here are four ways in which a lack of mourning can show up in a person's life if not properly addressed:

1. **Overworking or Overachieving:**

   Submerging into work and achievements is a way to avoid our pain and hide the depression. Work can bring satisfaction, success, and fulfillment but it also can create a distraction from dealing with the pain of loss. Many people seek affirmation and approval through work, performance, and promotion. So, it is not uncommon to find a person submerging himself into work after losing a loved one. If this is you, then take time to reflect on how to have a more balanced life in which you are not overworking, and give thought to dealing with the depression so that you can have a healthier and more balanced lifestyle.

2. **Dysfunctional Relationships**

   It's possible that when we lose a mother, the unresolved processing of the pain caused by her passing could make it difficult to connect in romantic relationships. The uncertainty and lack of being able to control the relationship and person may cause us to push away the people that we love and that love us.

3. **Grumpiness or Moodiness**

   Mood swings and being grumpy may be a by-product of our depression. The inconsistent mood swings could be triggered at any moment for various reasons. *Unresolved pain will create unpleasant attitudes.* Decide today that you will take action to address the moods that you may have that may be negatively affecting your life and the relationships that you have around you.

4. **Sexual Intimacy**

   The desire for or capability to engage in sexual intimacy can be affected if you do not grieve properly. A person can have a decrease in sexual interest or have an increase in unhealthy sexual relationships. If they are in a relationship, it can discourage a partner from being sexually intimate, greatly increase sexual intimacy, or cause other problems within the relationship. This, in turn, can add fuel to other issues or problems within the relationship with the significant other. In order to receive healing, save a relationship, and live in our new normal, we must be open to talk about how grief can affect the ability to be intimate.

The Trap of Suicidal Thoughts

First, let me start by saying that if you are contemplating suicide or are thinking of taking your own life, contact a professional. You have a purpose and a life to live. The haunting thoughts of suicide can come to any person. Despite our loss, this season is temporary. There is a great plan for our lives, and we should embrace every opportunity to live it to the fullest.

Defeating depression in the season of loss involves changing our mindset, perspective, and confession of the situation into a well-balanced, healthy conclusion. When my mother went home to be with the Lord, I really wished that she could have been a survivor. I wanted to be able to take the Breast Cancer walk with her because she had beaten the cancer. Though my mother's life was prolonged longer than the original diagnosis, I would have liked the outcome to be different, but the road traveled to support, pray, and stand in faith was not in vain.

4 Positive Actions To Destroy Depression

> *"Finally, brothers and sisters, whatever is true, whatever is noble, whatever is right, whatever is pure, whatever is lovely, whatever is admirable—if anything is excellent or praiseworthy—think about such things."*
> Philippians 4:8

In Philippians, the Apostle Paul wrote about how we should think. Our thought process affects every area of our lives. If we are positive thinkers, then we can have positive results. However, if we think negatively we will have negative results. I did not want to let go of my grief or my pain. For me, letting go of my pain would mean admitting that my mother was gone. The fear of what was on the other side kept me bound to the depression. I had to become intentional about thinking about the good things in my life to overcome this despair to live a better life. By faith and prayer, I was able to overcome that tough time. Here are some things that you can do to overcome depression after losing a mother:

1. **Positive Thinking:**

    Only think of the things that are positive and true in your life. Think about the things that are in the Word of God, and the things that God said about you that were true.

2. **Positive Confession:**

    Create positive confessions that will help you to move forward in a healthy way during your grief process. The more that you confess positive things, the better your thought process becomes and your life. \

3. **Positive Believing:**

   Believe in things that are positive. Have faith in God for your deliverance and through your time loss. Believe that He can help you.

4. **Positive Praying:**

   Pray and ask God to help you and give you strength. As you go through this journey, be sure to pray about your pain, your deliverance, and your future.

Remember, you can do this! You can overcome depression! You do not have to be bound to negative thoughts and ideas. There are brighter days ahead and those days can start now if you allow it. Your future is bright! Continue in your journey in a positive way.

Destroying Depression With Faith And Prayer
Making It Personal

Are you experiencing deep sadness or loss of hope? Take 15 minutes to write free style about all of the positive things in your life. Don't over-think it; just write freely as it comes to your mind. Based upon the things on that list, create a confession that you can recite daily to help you to think of positive things. Keep it in a place that you would see often like the refrigerator, bathroom, or in your bedroom so that you can confess daily.

Wearing The Mask

There is a common trap that many of us step into, called "wearing the mask." This trap does not allow for us to be authentic to who we are and to our journey. The issue of wearing a mask can also be found in faith-based circles. This where even believers act as though everything is fine and that nothing is wrong with them because of their faith in God. The masks that we wear cover our pain and hinder us from being human. Being enslaved to wearing a mask could have just as harsh of a chokehold on our happiness and joy as being enslaved to actual issues we face.

Pain does not have a religious denomination or affiliation. Pain is only loyal to causing affliction and more pain. Acting as though nothing has taken place in our lives keeps us from our deliverance, and it can stifle our growth towards reaching our God-given purpose. True deliverance happens when we are real. It happens when we truly recognize that God is the sole source of our healing, grace, love, forgiveness, and deliverance. When we surrender the need to look a certain way and please other people, we can receive total transformation and healing. Our purpose becomes attainable. Our vision becomes crystal clear. If you are wearing a mask, I want to encourage you to remove the mask and to be real with where you are so that you can receive your healing. I promise you that God will not let you down. He will catch you. He wants to be there for you. He already knew that this would happen in your life, so He made preparations to be there for you. He sent His Son Jesus for times like this. He sent Jesus to close the gap so that He Himself could connect with you, by the Holy Spirit, and so you would never be alone or remain trapped in the snare of despair.

Remember, we are talking about our mother. It is acceptable to be authentic and true to your journey during the time of grief recovery.

Wearing The Mask
Making It Personal

After reading this section, in which areas of your life do you believe that you are wearing a mask? Could you recall a time when you became stuck in your journey? What challenges have you experienced with wearing the mask or being stuck? What are the most important things you would like to accomplish by becoming unstuck? What would becoming unstuck make you feel or do differently?

Motherless Child In Crisis

"One of the hardest things I am struggling with right now is accepting that I am a motherless child. I don't want to be. But I know that whoever and whatever I am is not by accident. I know that He will watch over me and protect me, but I need to pull through this tough season. Who am I now that I am a motherless child? Father, I am in critical condition. I am in crisis mode. I am spinning all over the place. Help me understand who I am."
~ Journal Entry

Motherless Child In Crisis

In order to understand the power of your transformation, you must first understand the depth of your conflict and pain. *Transformation requires change and effort, but it is a work that will reward you in the end.* Obtaining your transformation will depend on how well you confront your inner struggles, starting from the initial point of your pain and finding fulfillment in the manifestation of your promise.

In my story, one of my inner struggles was centered completely on the reality that I was a motherless child, who had to learn how to cope with life without having a mother. I felt abandoned by her whether it was her fault or not, and I was angry about it. **I grappled with feeling unequipped to make it without her as a woman, mother, and wife.** I only knew that I must pull through. Several of my friends had already experienced this kind of loss. I found myself resenting many elders in the previous generation who I believed failed to step up to support in the time of need. I had unanswered questions and had so many turning pieces in my life that it was becoming exhausting and overwhelming. It seemed like I had hit rock bottom and was at an all-time low.

I was surprised by the reactions and responses that I had received by others after my mother passed away. My world at the time was full of drama, family misunderstandings, lawsuits over assets, unsupportive individuals, apprehension about motherhood, and a marriage in the midst of a tough season.

I was a motherless child in crisis.

Lord, I need you!

One day, in particular, I was sitting in our family room watching television, and my daughter came up to me and said, "Mommy, I love you." Then she proceeded to kiss me on both cheeks and forehead, which was the same way I would kiss her. The smile on her face was heart-warming. She was hoping to cheer me up. I hugged her tight and then gazed into her eyes and said, *"Did an angel send you over here to mommy?"* She smiled at me, and I held her so tight. I squeezed her so hard. In that moment, with tears running down my face, I cried unto the Lord. I said:

"Father, I need you! I need you. Help me find my joy. Make me into a happy mother. I can't do this on my own. Heal me! So that my child and future children will know what it means to have joy, be happiness, and healing, even if they go through a tough time. They will have their own unique purpose to win, lead, and make a difference. Please help me to be an example of how to travel that path the best way I can, and most importantly, to point them to Christ."

In Jesus' name!

I cried over her shoulder so she wouldn't see me. Then I wiped my face and pulled away from our hug. I smiled at her and told her that I loved her. The love for my daughter was what God used to pull me through. I did not have enough love for myself at the time. My little girl ignited hope inside of me. My truth was that I wanted things back to the way that they were before my mother had passed away. I did not want a new normal or for it to be as the old saints would say for my *"mom to dance with angels."* I wanted my mother here with me. I missed everything about my mother. I missed my irreplaceable mother.

Perhaps my story is similar to yours. Perhaps you are stuck in limbo between your anger and abandonment finding it difficult to transition into your transformation because of the pain you are experiencing in the moment, and the fear of what is on the other side. Whether you are a man or woman, you may be a motherless child in crisis and miss your own irreplaceable mother. It is essential to cry unto the Lord in prayer in the most authentic and heartfelt way.

In this season, do not be concerned about the opinions of others. You do not have to be in a church building to start your transformation. Transformation can start and manifest in a living room, just as it can in the four walls of a church building. As believers, "we" are the church and we carry the Holy Spirit with us. I have never seen religion save or deliver anyone, but I have witnessed the power of Jesus Christ through a personal relationship with Him transform a person's life from the depths of despair to a place of purpose that is filled with hope, joy, and peace.

Was Praying For My Mother A Good Thing?

A person of faith may wonder if praying for their mom was a good thing, or whether God valued or heard their prayers. This question can come up when there has been prayer for the mother's healing from cancer, but she did not receive the healing that they would have liked. I too had this question.

Praying for our mother, or any person is always a good thing and is never a wasted prayer.

I remember when the doctors first told us about my mother's tumor. I immediately began to pray about it. I called my church family and all of my prayer warriors and asked them to pray for my mother's healing. I was fortunate to have friends of all races, ethnicities, and doctrinal backgrounds who genuinely loved and cared for me as a sister in Christ, so it was a no-brainer for everyone that I notified to get into agreement about my mother. The only question that they had was, "What are we believing for and what is our assignment?" Halleluiah! The doctors didn't think she would live long from the initial diagnosis, but I was determined that we would turn that situation around. We were heavily committed to going to war on that tumor through prayer and daily confessions.

It was a difficult time emotionally, spiritually, and physically. Undergoing the breast cancer treatment process is very exhausting for the whole family. There are so many gaps that need to be filled and support that is needed throughout the chemo process. It took its toll emotionally because we were witnessing someone we cared about struggle right before our eyes and we could not take the pain away.

Praying for those we love is actually the *best* use of our time. A true prayer warrior puts their heart into prayer and lay it all on the altar. In the midst of the storm, it is best to stay focused on the promise and to avoid distractions. We should stay positive, and give everything that we have to faith and prayer. The Word of God says,

"The prayer of a righteous person is powerful and effective."
James 5:16

When righteous people pray, there is much power. Even if you did not have the best relationship with God at the time, but had a heartfelt prayer for your mother, He heard you. Christ is not a judge waiting to count all of your wrongdoings when you need Him most. Ideally, we would like to know of Him before those times, but if it takes those moments to come to Him then so be it. He still welcomes us with warm arms. God's not surprised by our prayers, responses, or fears. Therefore, be encouraged about praying for your mother whether it was your first time praying, if you hadn't prayed in a while, or if you were a seasoned prayer warrior. Your prayers were meaningful not only for the person who you were praying for but also in the work that began in you. Your prayers have brought power, and they will never be wasted. Even if the outcome was not what you would have liked for it to be or what you intended, it does not mean your prayers lacked power.

Our mothers are heroes. There is absolutely nothing to be ashamed of or to be sad about when someone as amazing as an irreplaceable mother has transitioned and is surrounded by love and prayer. Therefore, be confident and encouraged if you prayed for your mother's healing. Take solace in knowing that you gave the best gift that anyone could give. You gave the gift of prayer. By praying for your mother, you took actions of faith and love towards her.

Motherless Child In Crisis
Making It Personal

What actions are you willing to commit to for your transformation? When you think of your transformation, what do you see in your life? After reading this chapter, what positive things do you now see have come from the prayers that you prayed for your mother?

Being The Strong One

I remember the drive home after we received the news about how fatally our mother's disease had progressed, and my first thought was to fix it. I thought to myself, "*I know what I will do. I will fix it.*" I could not entertain anything other than her receiving her healing. I was still processing what the doctors said. "*Did he just say that my mother was dying and that there was nothing we could do? How could this be?*" I was the oldest daughter and was determined to fix everything. I kept a hard exterior so that people could not see what I was really going through. I did not want to deal with any of the negativity or naysayers in that time. My focus was on the cure and getting through the situation.

I was angry with myself.

As unhealthy as it may sound, I blamed myself for my mom's passing for a long time because I could not save her. I could not fix it. I used to feel as though I was this woman who had it all together. I had my struggles, sure. I blamed myself for not being able to be as available as I felt I ought, and for not checking in on the doctors more. I blamed myself for not taking more authority over the situation. I took myself down a dark path because I kept replaying in my mind what I could have done differently. The answer was simple—nothing! But that did not stop me from thinking that way.

I thought I was the strong one. After my mother died, I realized that I was not as strong or in faith as I thought. In reality, I was being controlling to make sure things stuck together. I was placing all hope on myself and relying on my own strength. On the inside, I was a scared little girl who loved her mother. I thought that when my mother died, I would have just fallen apart to a place of no return. Something amazing was revealed when she passed away: a moment that I expected to cause me to crumble under pressure caused me to grow in my faith instead. I noticed that I did not have any control—and I was okay. I was perfectly fine. The apocalypse did not take place. It was in that moment that I realized that I was stronger than I thought, and my faith in God was what needed to be strong. Not faith in myself. My confidence increased because I began to stop needing to control and understand every little detail and focus on the ones that would add value to others.

I understood that my need to fix everything was unhealthy. I just did not know what to do. I had been with my mother since she was young. My mother and father were married at 20 years old, and they had me at 21 years old. We all basically grew up together. I remember the years throughout her twenties and into her thirties. My mother wasn't even 40 years old when she attended my high school graduation. I am three and a half years older than my sister right under me; I am almost seven years older than my youngest sister and almost 11 years older than my youngest brother. The role that I had growing up was primarily to take care of everyone else. I was around when my parents were learning how to be parents, and getting situated in life.

Typically, my role in the house as the oldest girl was to take care of my younger siblings while my parents were at work. I was responsible for making sure everyone completed his or her homework and household chores. Many times, I felt as though I was a like a third parent because of the way family duties would be placed on me. I saw and knew many things that went on in the house. My younger siblings did not see all of the things that I did in my parents' early and middle years. Because I saw and knew as much as I did, I believe it made it even harder for me to let go or to show my true feelings.

There came a point in time that I had to learn to let it go, and that it was not my fault. If something happened to me, the last thing I would want any of my children to think is that my passing was their fault. I wouldn't want any of my children to carry such a burden, as I am sure that many other mothers do not. As a mom, I would want my children to know that I loved them and that was what mattered most. Even if one of my children made a mistake, I still would not blame them. I would not care anyway and would forgive them. There is not any way that I could be in heaven, a place of perfection, worship, and glory and hold a grudge against anyone, let alone one of my children.

Be Human

I made the error of not allowing myself to be human like everyone else. I was busy keeping up with my affairs. I was still trying to make sure everything was okay with everyone else, but I did not take time for myself. Be okay with who you are. Don't think that you need to be the strong one and in control. It is okay to grieve. You don't have to be that "perfect person" in this season of your life.

Be okay with not being okay.

It is okay to be upset for a while but just don't stay that place. Be sure to work through your issues in a way that is healthy. We don't always know how to properly place our anger or blame. As we sort through the emotions and situations in our lives, let's be sure to have balance and avoid being the person who tries to act like they have it all together.

If you are anything like me or resonate with this part of my story, then know that it is not your fault. So many of us can suffer unnecessarily from blaming ourselves or feeling responsible for taking care of someone. It is so important to realize that you are not alone. We do not always know why things may happen, but as believers, we should never be ashamed or upset about being there for someone and praying about it. We do not pray simply to receive. We pray out of a relationship with our heavenly Father through Christ. The answers to our prayers may not come in the package that we thought that they would. Our prayers are answered in many ways. Decide today that you start the journey to release your anger and to live a life that is free from the bondage of being the strong one.

Being The Strong One
Making It Personal

What are your thoughts about God being sovereign and in control? What positive things can you begin to think about regarding your prayers for your mother? Are you dealing with being mad at God? If so, write down your thoughts and why you feel the way that you do. What would you like to see improved in your thinking about your situation?

Peace For The Abandoned And Angry

"It's not fair. I hate cancer! I really hate cancer! This is the hardest thing I have had to endure, but I know that God will get the glory. My mom was the strongest woman I ever knew. She taught me so much in her life and by how she passed away. She would want me to live on and be happy. So do I."

~ *Journal entry*

It's Not Fair

My mother was my greatest teacher. She taught me amazing lessons about life and people. She was an example of grace and honor. Sometimes it doesn't seem real that your mother has passed away until you go through it yourself. Life goes on, and it does not slow down just because you had a tragedy or trauma.

As mentioned, during the time of my mother's health challenge with breast cancer, our entire family was engaged in her journey and completely supportive of her. Everyone sowed their own talents, gifts, and treasures according to what they could do in their own life. There was so much going on such as doctor's appointments, surgeries, and consultations. I believe we were all on autopilot. However, if asked whether we would do it again, I believe that we would all respond with a resounding "YES!" I don't regret one moment supporting my mother in her health challenge because she was an instrumental part of my life and had done so much for me. During the process, I handled all of my mother's estate, finances, and paperwork. I was the eldest and was the most responsible when it came to finances. Many other family members also had valuable roles during the process because of their shared love for her.

My mother had to continue working despite having cancer. This added pressure to her treatment process, but she was committed to going to every doctor's and physical therapy appointment with a smile, which was admirable to everyone who witnessed her journey. My father was amazingly supportive and volunteered to go with her to all of her doctor's appointments when he was available. Though my parents were divorced, he really stepped up to make sure that my mother did not go through the cancer process alone. It was a very admirable act that we would always appreciate on her behalf. All of us had our own roles, but the greatness of that season was that everyone united on that one issue without question, second-guessing, or misunderstanding.

It doesn't matter what stage of a person's life they are in when their mother gets ill or passes away. It could happen when a mother is young or when they are old; nevertheless, we would never want them to go. If we could have it our way, we would have them live with us forever. I've learned that some people get more time and some get less. Others may not have had the experience of having their mother in their lives at all.

It may seem like it is unfair, that the odds were stacked against you, and that this is not the right thing. It may seem like you did not get what you wanted. Rest assured, that what appears to be a stumbling block will one day turn into a stepping-stone. Unjust as it seems today, there will be moments of clarity that will shine through your times of cloudy understanding to give you hope, comfort, and motivation.

How Does God Feel About This?

Personally, I believe that God is not happy with our pain. He did not create us to give us this pain of sickness and disease. Based upon the Word of God in the book of Genesis, we received this pain from the fall of man, when Adam and Eve sinned in the Garden of Eden. The Garden of Eden was perfect. There was not any sickness, disease, or sin. However, because of the sin of man, God had to remove Adam and Eve from the Garden of Eden and separate Himself from mankind. Thus, after the fall, He had to separate Himself from the sinful nature of mankind, a creation that He made after His own image. Not forgetting the obvious separation of when Jesus went through our redemption process. God was separated from His Son, Jesus, through that process. Jesus thought that God the Father had forsaken Him while He was on the cross, but He did not. Therefore, God understands our pain of separation and connects with our situation. He isn't far removed from us and distant from our problems. Sometimes, it is hard to understand where God is with all of the things we are going through. He never intended for us to endure the trials of this world as we are now. In the Word of God, God says that death is an enemy and it is an enemy that He plans to destroy.

For he must reign until he has put all his enemies under his feet.
The last enemy to be destroyed is death.
1 Corinthians 15:25-26

This passage of scripture is encouraging for us because it can get cloudy sometimes to know where God is when we experience a difficult loss such as losing our mother especially if we prayed for her healing. In this scripture, He said that the last enemy that He will destroy is death. This scripture gave me comfort because it placed death as God's enemy. He made it clear that He will one day wipe out death, sickness, and disease. When I read this scripture, I then started to have hope. I had hope because He truly was not a God who left me, but a God who will one day deliver a fierce blow against the devil and destroy all of his plans of death, disease, and destruction. He will put an end to all sickness and disease in the world. Cancer will be no more! Pain will be no more! Motherless children will be no more! No one will have to experience this type of loss again, and we will be reunited with our loved ones!

Halleluiah! I began to praise God through my tears. My deliverance had not come yet when I first read this passage, but I gained a little more hope through knowing that my Father was on my side and understood my situation. His understanding and empathy is shown even further in the following scripture:

> *"For we do not have a high priest who is unable to empathize with our weaknesses, but we have one who has been tempted in every way, just as we are—yet he did not sin."*
> *Hebrews 4:15*

Therefore, as we recover from our grief, we can live in peace knowing that we have a God who is connected and relates to us. I pray that this scripture gives you hope and sheds some light on where God is in your life for your situation. God is on your side. He is not your enemy. He is not out to get you or hurt you. One day, we all will receive justice against our enemy the devil, when God will put an end to death, sickness, disease, and pain once and for all.

Why Didn't God Heal Her?

> *"Trust in the Lord with all your heart and lean not on your own understanding; in all your ways submit to him, and he will make your paths straight."*
> Proverbs 3:5-6

If I could have a moment of transparency, I was upset with God after my mother passed away. Yes, the born again, Spirit-filled believer was angry and angry with God at that. Shortly after my mother's passing, I did not know how to deal with my emotions. I recall reciting one of my favorite sayings, which was: "As long as I have Jesus and my momma I will be okay." It was really hard for me to understand why my mother had to die. When she died, I felt as though I was let down by God. In that moment, for the first time ever, I felt that I did not have Jesus or my mother. I knew that it was going to be a long, hard road for us without having a mother in our lives.

This is a common question for people to ask, whether they identify as being a believer in Christ or not. It is a universal question regardless of the religious background that a person may come from, especially if the circumstances that they are left behind to cope with are unfavorable. We may ask questions like, *"Why didn't God heal her?"* or *"Where are you, God?"* We make the common mistake in believing that healing has not occurred or is not taking place. Like I mentioned, our healing is not always physical. God is sovereign no matter whether we understand how or why things happen or not.

> *"Our God is in heaven; he does whatever pleases him."*
> Psalm 115:3

Therefore, taking comfort in His sovereignty will anchor us in the fact that there is always something working in our best interest. We simply must trust and believe, even if it's a small step of faith.

God Is In Control

Why do some people get to live old and others die young? Well, I realized that no matter what time they leave, God is still in control. His sovereignty is what we need to trust. No matter when a mother passes away, her children must always know that He is sovereign and that He will protect them. Even though we may not like the outcome of what we are dealing with, we must accept that everything that happens has a divine purpose.

> **It's Not Fair**
> **Making It Personal**
>
> What are your thoughts about God being sovereign and in control? What positive things can you begin to think about regarding your prayers for your mother? Are you dealing with being mad at God? If so, write down your thoughts and why you feel the way that you do. What would you like to see improved in your thinking about your situation?

> *"Dear Mommy,*
> *I was hurt because of some of the decisions you made with my father,*
> *in my life, and in leaving me. I am angry because I feel that you*
> *have abandoned me and left me here alone."*
> ~ Journal entry

Hidden Anger

Who would have thought that it is possible to be angry with a person who has passed away? I had to be honest with myself: deep down inside, I was angry with my mother. Even though this was a woman who I adored more than anything, I had issues with her. I was upset about her decision to keep all of her children in the dark about the severity of her breast cancer condition for so long because all of us were adults. It was her decision, but if I were honest with myself, I did not like it.

Over the years, I've met women who have been diagnosed with cancer or another illness who have asked me my opinion about whether or not they should share the true condition of their cancer with their children. I share with them that if it is possible to do so, and then yes. Allowing your children and loved ones to take care of you and love on you will help your loved ones through the journey and live on if something were to ever happen with you.

I was also angry with my mother for keeping me in the dark about the issues and concerns with my father's difficulty with connecting with me. My father and I did not always get along, and he did not accept a role in the breakdown of our relationship despite my complaints about our relationship. It appeared that my mother withheld the truth from me and held back important information about our breakdown in an attempt to protect me from the truth about my relationship with my father. But her decision to protect me from the truth ended up hurting me even more down the road. In my mind, I believed that she underestimated my strength and maturity to understand my situation and ability to handle the truth about my father. I desired that she had trusted me at the time. My mother, as with many other mothers, engaged in an unhealthy and unwanted juggling act of attempting to keep peace and the family together, by avoiding the core issues of the breakdown of our relationship. Because this breakdown was never addressed during her life, the breakdown continued over when she passed away, and I was upset about it. It was a defining moment in my grief recovery to come to terms that I had an issue with my mother. It was one of the key components that I needed to address in order to getting over to the other side of my grief.

For some of us, there comes a point where we have to have a grown-up moment and accept that our mother's were *just as much someone else's lover as she was our mother*. I came to that very realization with my own mother. I recognized that she fell in love with a man, got married, had a family, and wanted to have the man that she loved along with the children that she loved.

I may not have liked all of my mother's choices, but she was an adult with her own life. It is not required that I like or accept her choices. It is more important that I recognize that her choices are a reflection of her own life.

When I really settled on the decision that I wanted to heal and recover from my pain of loss and forgive others, I had to be open to seeing the good and the bad of my mother as well. I could not place my mother up on a pedestal of perfection. At times, it can be easy to be upset with everyone else, but it takes real self-reflection and humility to acknowledge that some of our pain and hurt may have come from the person who has passed away, even the mother who was so important to us.

I encourage you today, that if you have anger against your mother that has passed away or the people that may be left behind like your father, or any family member, you are not alone. There may be have been decisions and lessons made during your mother's life that may be hindering you in your current season. The obstacles that you may have encountered with getting unstuck to get your healing may be in part due to the choices that were made by the deceased, not necessarily that you did anything wrong. If you truly want to receive your healing, be prepared to face those truths, so that you can receive your healing in your recovery process.

Building A Tribe

Our support system was broken. There was not a succession plan given on how to be there for the children in terms of responsibilities when our mother passed away. This led me to become more intentional about the friends and tribe that I began to build as a wife and young mother. I began to become more intentional about sharing my vision and dreams with people around me about my desires for my children's future, the type of people that I would like for them to become, and the lifestyles they should live. My husband and I were always good about planning for the future, but we took extra measures to make sure that our children's futures were protected if something were to ever happen to us. We partnered with other family and friends and began to make agreements about how we would check up on each other's children in the event something happened to us. Overall, I wanted to make sure to the best of my ability that there was a support structure in place for them, and that I had good friends in my circle.

Lost Without A Parent

"I lost a father when I lost my mom. I felt like had a double loss. But he wasn't connected before she passed away. It is hard to process all of this loss all at once. It seems like everyone is passing away at the same time, or that people are dividing at the same time. When will this situation let up? Why do I have to approach this alone without a parent? Father, help me and be the father that I need in this season. Please fill in the gaps and show me the way in this journey."

~ Journal Entry

This next part of my story details some of the toughest aspects of coping with my mother's death, specifically in regard to my experience with my father and siblings after she died. The pain this experience caused me was immense, and I am aware I may have caused pain in return. I couldn't understand why God would have me go through something like this so soon after losing my irreplaceable mother, but in the end, it looked like He had a plan for me in it all.

My father was a family man and hard worker. My parents worked hard to provide for our family and to have fun activities. As mentioned, my father and I had a complicated relationship with its ups and downs. We had great family moments in a group, and he was physically present and active in my life. However, we did not see eye to eye with each other one on one. Many people said we were two peas in a pod and had similar qualities, which was very true. What was also true was that my father and I struggled with making a real connection emotionally or spiritually as father and daughter. My father was always there for me as a provider, protector, and advisor to the physical care of me as his daughter. Life was not always easy for us, but both of my parents always did their best to provide for us. One of our biggest issues between us, I believed, was that my father did not know me as a person, and what he believed that he knew about me was nothing like me at all. He did not know me as a person, young girl, woman, or as a Christian. Deep down inside I wanted more from my father. I wanted a better relationship with him that involved more than just the work or business relationship. My friends at school began to go to a local church called Word of Faith and invited me to the youth ministry. I wasn't saved at the time and did not understand their zeal for their faith, but I knew it seemed interesting. I never heard anyone talk about Jesus the way that they did. They spoke of Him like He was a friend and father, which was something that I was missing in the context that they spoke.

My father invited me to Perfecting Church and suggested that I attend one of the services. He occasionally attended their church services and almost always went to their New Years Eve services. He wasn't a member, but he really liked the pastor. He said that the pastor was down to earth and he could understand his teachings. I had visited the church a few times, and it was exactly as my father described. The pastor's teaching was relatable, charismatic, and connected with what I was going through. I didn't understand everything he preached about, but I sensed that I needed what was he was offering at the altar call. I did not completely understand all of the details about the gospel, but I did know that I wanted eternal life with God. I sensed the tug on my heart to go to the altar for a few services but was afraid to follow the urge to go to the front of the church, so I did not move from the pew. One Sunday, it happened! I answered the tug on my heart and went to the altar before the pastor even completed the invitation to the congregation to accept Jesus Christ in my heart as Lord and Savior! I stood at the altar alone, looking around aimlessly. In that moment, I don't know what to expect. I don't know if there was going to be a light from heaven that was going to beam down or that an angel was going to come down to minister to me. I have attended church services in other churches in the past and went to various programs, but I never heard the gospel broken down before until now. A woman noticed that I was standing at the altar alone, and walked up to me. She immediately grabbed and hugged me. *How did she know to do that?* I thought. Because I was happy that she did. As soon as she hugged me, I fell into her arms and cried in her arms during the rest of the pastor's invitation. I hoped that she had another blouse because I got all of my tears out on her shoulder on that day. Tears flowed and flowed from my eyes as I released my pains and burdens over to the Lord. I felt a huge weight and burden lifted from my shoulders as if a ton of bricks were taken away from me. I was 17 ½ years old during my senior year of high school when I gave my life to Christ. The service was amazing and life-changing. Shortly after making the decision to give my life to Christ, there was a noticeable increase in conflict with the relationships around me. However, I did not know that it was due to my decision to give my life to Christ at the time because I was still a baby Christian. I was unaware of how to fight or that I was even apart of a battle during that time. I was the only one in my family who was saved or born again at the time. Little did I know, that I was also the only one on the trajectory to try to learn about and live for God. I didn't know at the time, but the decision to follow Christ would set the stage for conflict in the future, even when my mother became sick and passed away.

I was excited about going to school to tell my friends about the decision that I made. When I went to school the next day, I told them about how I gave my life to Christ, and they all cheered, hugged me, and hollered like they were in a basketball championship game! It was welcoming and hilarious at the same time. For the first time, I felt like I was at home and in the right place. I felt like they were my kind of people and crowd that I wanted to be around. It wasn't because they were all the best Christians either. As a matter of fact, some were from broken backgrounds, first-generation saved, and dysfunctional situations just like me, but knew that they loved Christ, and wanted to learn more about Him. We had a few in the group that came from Christian backgrounds and may have had more experiences with the gospel, but they were all really nice and we lovingly designated them to be our leaders and share information. For the first time, in a long time, I felt like this was where I needed to be.

On the other hand, when I shared the news of my salvation with my parents, it was not so well received. I received more of an "oh really" type of response from them. My father was a down to earth person but did not relate to my journey of faith very well. At times, that journey of discovery and growth could have been in the shadows because I travelled it alone for the most part. My efforts to learn about Christ through attending small groups, youth group and events at the church were overlooked, dismissed, discounted, and dishonored. This hurt me a lot, especially with my father. This was an important part of my life, and I could not share it with him. I would watch other kids and witness how their parents would celebrate their faith achievements and congratulate them on walking with God, but for me, there were no such celebrations or acknowledgements of my attempts to achieve highly personal growth. If I were to volunteer at a senior citizen's home, youth group, or community event for church or to simply serve, there was not any positive reinforcement or affirmation in that area of my life from my family. Most of the time, I participated in those events and walked that journey with my friends at church. As time went on, my church family almost became my family. My god-sisters and god-brothers became closer to me than my own biological family at times. My god-sisters and sister-friends, who is another name for best friends, were my rock and supported me with prayer, encouragement, and rebuke throughout the years, as mentioned earlier. Though I was always grateful for it, I believe that I wished that I could share that journey with my own family, especially with my father. Our relationship started to get worse. He hurt me, and I am sure he had been hurt by me. From my observation, our broken relationship only created more resentment and contention in a very unhealthy way. Though he and I were father and daughter, there were times were our disagreements were more like brother and sister or husband and wife. He made the decision to only connect to my flaws, sin, and mistakes; and was adamant about pointing them out at any opportunity that he received. This caused many arguments between others and us because his behavior traits disturbed me and others copied them. I believe it caused me to lean closer towards my relationship with God as Father. I wanted to know God as a Father and understand what He was about. I believe it also caused me to hold back a little on my relationship with God at first because I had a hard time understanding how God could be all of the great things that my biological father wasn't, but I am to refer to Him as "Abba Father."

From an early age, our relationship was a mixed bag. In one moment, he would teach me about business and how to operate in the world so that I would not get taken advantage of, but then in the next moment he was coming against about how badly I was doing or holding a grudge against me. My father had some good qualities that could not be discounted. I believe that is one of the reasons I always worked hard at doing well in school, business, and learning about the world, was to get his approval. It was also a way for me to spend time with him, even if we were fighting. When he was in the zone of business and work, he was a wealth of knowledge, wisdom, and fun. Yet there were many qualities that I needed and desired as a daughter that he did not possess nor desired to acquire. I needed a connection. I needed someone to be concerned about me and to see me for who I am. As time went on, it was clear that he and I simply never cultivated that type of emotional connection in a way that was healthy and that I needed.

My father has always been there for me in times of trouble. I had and have no doubt that if I ever was in trouble, he would help me. Our struggles were centered with knowing and being able to assist me with matters of the soul. Because of this conflict, internally I could not understand why God would allow my mother, who loved me unconditionally, prayed for me, and genuinely cared for me would be taken away from me, and I would be left behind with a parent who did not know how or could not love me, as I needed. This conflict caused a lot of pain in my grief recovery because my father could not even feel my pain when my mother passed away, which was reflected in the fruit of our relationship after my mother passed away. He could not connect with me in her life, and could not connect with me after her passing.

I believe that many misunderstandings that appeared when my mother passed away started well before her home going. My mother's home going uncovered deep-rooted issues that were there. Perhaps you can relate to that story in your own journey after your mother passed away. Maybe there were issues in the background that you were unaware of that began to play itself out soon after your irreplaceable mother went home to be with the Lord. In my personal story, there were times that my mother was accused of showing favoritism towards me or allowing for me to do what I wanted. This assumption began to architect a division between me and family members, separate us emotionally and spiritually, and create underlining resentment that rung so deep that it seemed almost impossible for those caught in its web to get out of it. This led to very hurtful acts towards me without punishment or concern for me, after she passed away. Unfortunately, my father played a role in the discord, and escalated many problems by not holding all parties within our family and friend circle equally accountable to their actions. For example, there could be certain situations could happen to me and there would not be any consequences or fall out for what I experienced, but if the situation were reversed, he would attempt to punish me and hold resentment against me for doing it, even if it weren't true. Nonetheless, he never held resentment or took issue with anything that anyone ever did with or said to me, which was hurtful to me. During her life, my mother attempted to be a peacemaker and wanted everyone to get along, but she did not make the proper attempts to work through the issues. By not addressing the issues, my mother allowed them to continue.

Once my mother passed away, the conflict with the family and friend circles heightened like never before. There were destructive relationships had erupted into vicious battles over estates and control. The hidden issues of the past spilled over into the season of bereavement when my mother passed away. As the parent left behind, my father was emotionally disconnected to how all of these actions impacted me as a grieving daughter, wife, or mother with a young family. Therefore, he could not support me during that time.

I share this because these types of conflicts played a role in my recovery process. I did not know it at the time, but there were wounds and issues that were being piled on on top of the issue of grief. I came to conclusion that these types of actions and experiences would affect my life and my healing process. I was not a saint in any of my relationships, but some of the continual division impacted my ability to heal properly. It was a though I trying to heal one scar and as I was applying medicine to the wound, another scratch would appear. Thus, it began to become difficult to get the healing I desired because I was in a state of turmoil and confusion.

Perhaps there are parts of my story that resonates with you, your family, friends, or someone you know. They may be different characters, a different set, and maybe a different plot, but it has the same storyline. There is a person that you may have had conflict with during your mother's life, and it increased when they passed away. Perhaps you discovered that there were those around you that may have had resentment or animosity against you because of the deceased. To your surprise, you may have discovered that it was those that were closest to you. Like me, maybe you recognized that you have hidden anger against your mother because of the choices that she has made. During the time of grief recovery, it is important to realize that true healing may not take the form that we are used to but take the form in what is most needed. We must also identify what may be hindering our ability to get our healing so that we can move forward in a healthy way.

Hidden Anger
Making It Personal

After reading this chapter, do you consider yourself to be angry with a parent? If so, what things have caused you to be angry from your perspective? Is it hard to admit and acknowledge anger that you may have towards your mother? If so, why do you think that would be the case? Considering that our mothers and fathers are human like everyone else, what are some things that you now realize about who your parent is that you did not know before?

Why Can't We Be Friends?

Transformation can come from our hardest trials. Change occurs in tough places and situations. This is one reason why many people do not experience the transformation that they desire because they are unwilling to go through the trials or do the work that is required to obtain the change that they want in their life. Who likes family for friend drama? No one, right? There is nothing like family or friend drama after a significant person like a mother has passed away of any sickness, especially a long process such a cancer. There were times when my life looked like it was the hit movie *Soul Food*, where my mother was like the Big Momma character: when she passed, all of the kids left behind acted poorly. The drama was unreal. Her passing revealed a lot of resentment, unforgiveness, and jealousy in the background that many of us were unaware of. It also revealed the depth of pain and unforgiveness that members of the family carried with them. There were issues and conversations in the background that were never brought to my attention.

I loved my family. I took care of my mother's estate and financial affairs as always. I set up her retirement and insurance accounts made sure that all siblings and parties were taken care of in case of anything were to happen to her. I took care of the gaps of any expenses if needed, which was never an issue. But some members of the extended family did not like the fact that I managed the assets, even though I did so during her life and was the one who set them in place.

From the outside looking in, most would not have known the extent of the division and animosity. Underneath the surface, certain members created bonds between themselves to discuss issues they weren't happy about and united over what they agreed upon. It was interesting to see the perspective of many people unfold, as many of the opinions of family members did not surface until after my mother had passed away.

Did Anyone Notice?

I was our mother's oldest child. There were some who felt as though I had received more time from our mother and therefore they did not have to consider the affect of her passing as it related to me, in the same way that it affected my younger siblings. In certain situations, they acted as if I did not lose a mother as well. I had just as much control over my mother's passing as I did over my own birth, but they did not see it that way. Our mother would support me or provide for me in the background, but I was not made aware of these conversations of dissent until after she passed away. After these conversations with our mother, people would leave feeling angry *towards me*! I once asked, "*Did anyone notice that I was not in the room? Did anyone notice that I wasn't even around?*" Therefore, when I encountered my certain members at various times, I did not know what had gone on in the background and would get negative energy or comments out of the blue.

Family and friend drama is always hard after a key person like a mother figure has passed away. It can be especially painful if you discover how others may really feel about you once the person is gone. These types of discoveries happen primarily when the person, who passed away, such as a mother figure, was the glue person in the family who kept everyone in harmony. Once the mother has passed away, misunderstandings can populate. Misunderstandings can create a heartbreaking cycle of abuse and disrespect that if not addressed will continue to hurt those that are involved. Unfortunately, for a season, this was true in my case. Our pain clouded our thinking from the reality of who each other really were, who we dealing with, and how to process each other as individuals. I think it is easier for some people to be upset with others than to be upset with the deceased. In my case, I ensured that everyone in the family circle was taken care of through the financial planning and long-term plans when my mother went home to be with the Lord. They attributed those efforts to my mother instead. I had to learn how to look at things from a different point of view, even if I did not agree with it.

We have to accept that everyone has their own perspective about a situation after a person passes away and a method to address what they see. They may feel justified to do and say things that we believe is unjustifiable or doesn't make proper sense. The key in these type of situations is to acknowledge that it is not required that you share the same perspective as your family member or friend to gain your healing or freedom. Even though misunderstandings and division may hurt, it does not mean that you have to remain stuck in that pain. You can decide to live out your truth in faith and power.

Fuel To Fire

Fuel was added to the fire with lawsuits over property and assets. Family members were divided over these issues but little was done to de-escalate the issue. Relationships were completely shattered. I was disheartened by the fact that there was a lack of consideration on how these disagreements affect the children and young families. These were actions that I knew that my mother, if she were alive, would not allow or approve of. The lawsuits caused a wedge in so many relationships that it is unclear whether they can be repaired. Though there have been attempts to do so, the underlying issues still remain.

So there I was, a grieving young mother with young children, in court about assets, and a need to navigate through it all by faith. The lawsuits were hindering my ability to grieve, as I desired. Reflecting back, I don't think I realized just how much people will either try to take or destroy property, assets, and money once a person passes away.

Have you experienced drama or lawsuits over assets after your mother passed away? It can become draining and tough when the disputes happen after the person passes away. Lawsuits can divide a family, and typically they should be avoided. Only through prayer and faith can any person navigate through those troubled times, but the good news is that it is possible.

Invisible But Visible

Have you ever felt invisible? One of the main issues that I struggled with was being *visible*. I felt invisible when it came to my concerns or issues after my mother passed away. I desired to be seen and to have a voice when it came to the relationships around me. Recognizing that my feelings and concerns that were dismissed, dishonored, and disregarded was a hard truth to accept. I also had to accept that I played a role in some of the poor relationships that I had. I taught people how to treat me by allowing them to do so. I also did so by believing that I had to deal with it.

There are many perspectives to the situation when someone passes away. I believe that the perspective that we all have depends on the view of who the person was to us and who we were to them. Most of the time, we fail to try to see things from the other person's point of view because we see things from our own point of view or just from our own pain.

One of the most liberating truths that helped me with the recovery of my mother's passing was the truth that I was not invisible, but visible. Once I accepted that truth, I elevated on the road towards happiness and freedom.

Glue Person

When the "glue person" who holds a family together dies, the strands that held the group together may become broken. The division or revelation of the true nature of some relationships can appear unreal, but what is even worse is if the same lips that say that they love you, may internally despise you.

Are you struggling with division in your own circle after your glue person passed away? Are you struggling with being on the outside of the inner circle? Be authentic and be true to your self. During the time of grief, you may feel like you are on the outside, but you are still on the inside if you are in Christ. It may feel lonely or difficult at first, but the more you become comfortable about who you are, and accept the transition of the season of life you are in, the better you will be to position yourself to receive your healing.

Unique Perspectives

Discord of any sort is a difficult to navigate through after the passing of a mother. For me, one of the main casualties and consequences of losing a mother who is a glue person and having a broken relationship with my father was that my relationship with some of my sisters and brother would become more strained because of the stress of the funeral, the strained relationship with my dad, and the new normal that awaited us. We had always had a lot of fun together throughout the years and loved each other deep down inside. Our family always had the best family moments filled with vacations, Sunday dinners, and relaxing days at home firing up the BBQ grill making jokes about our week. *"Family first!"* was our motto. However, the pain of loosing a mother, along with the underlining division, took its toll on our relationships.

Unfortunately, the years of turmoil and division prior to our mother's passing prepared the stage and created an atmosphere of disheartening disrespect, dishonor, and disregard, which none us were happy about. It hit me especially hard because as I mentioned earlier in the book, I was nowhere close to the inner circle due to the path that I had taken my life and my faith. The earlier decisions that I made about my education, going to bible school, and volunteering the community afforded me with experiences and lessons that were not commonly shared in our dynamic. There was not any one else who shared or meditated on various lessons. Thus, when our mother passed away, we were not connected. They were all connected together and connected with my father. I was not connected due to the division and discord between my father, mother, and I. As I saw it, for them they all had commonalities in their journey and pain. They all had each other's backs, and they all backed each other up because they understood each other. Most importantly, there was not anyone else who could come to the table with any biblical or spiritual truths or insight to mend the situation. I believe that it was easier for me when I thought that it was just my father that I had to be mindful of, but I soon discovered that they were all common together, and I was not. The prayer, work, and life altering decisions that were made in how I would live my life played a role in how I was connected and supported after my mother passed away.

Perhaps, you feel disconnected as well. This may be because you too have made decisions in your life, about your faith, and your walk that placed you on the outside of the inner circle. If this is the case, know that you are not alone. In the background, they had their own experiences. While you were making decisions for your life, they were making decisions for theirs. Now that you are aware that there are different views, make the decision to walk in your truth so that you have the healing that you desire for your grief recovery.

Walk In Your Truth

Walking in your truth does not exempt you from any responsibility in the discord in your relationships. What it does is that it stops you from walking in someone else's truth, if their version includes negative energy or purpose-draining actions regarding you. One of the ways to address grief after a mother dies is by walking in the light of your story and experience without fear. You can't surround yourself with any level of negativity and expect to heal from the grief of losing someone as important as a mother figure in your life. The negative energy of others must be rejected so that you can receive your healing. Be honest about where you are, and be willing to communicate to others your truth even if that truth includes that you are not happy with their choices and desire that they respect your boundaries.

So walk in your truth. Sometimes disputes with family and friends may cause unpleasant issues, but continue to walk in your truth so that you can live the best life possible for you anyway. Pray for those relationships to heal and grow. If those relationships are too toxic, pray and ask God to give you the strength you need to separate from relationships that are no longer healthy for you and supports your quest for healing. For the relationships that are positive, pray and ask God to use those relationships to bring healing, restoration, and joy in your lives.

Why Can't We Be Friends?
Making It Personal

Have you experienced any discord since your mother passed away? Is there tension in relationships that were once close? How can you cope with your current situation and still get your healing? What steps could you take to ensure that you can move forward in a way that is healthy? Do you have strained relationships with anyone? If so, could you commit to praying for them?

Healing Through Forgiveness

"The pain is so real and so cold.
It has a crippling hook and grasp on my soul.
It's like an unwavering ache. I am ready to move on.
I must move on, but can I?
How can I be free from my pain, drama, and grief?
I am ready to be free. I need to let go once and for all--
everything and everyone that has hurt me."
~ Journal Entry

Freedom With Forgiveness

I wanted to be free but did not know how. I had chaos on every corner but did not know what it was. My heart was shattered into a million pieces. I was shattered. My heart was heavy. My sorrow was thick. Who would have thought that a person could be angry about being broken? But when you are brokayen, it affects your life, your thinking, and your joy. It's a detour on the road of your life. I did not realize at the time that it was a redirecting of my destiny.

I was sinking, and fast. The Titanic had nothing on me. How did I get to this point? What choices did I make to get here? Many times, when we go through things, God will use the difficult times to show us the poor choices, the poor actions, and the toxic people in our lives. Even when dealing with family and friends, we have to realize that some relationships may be toxic and unhealthy.

I allowed for the decisions of others to negatively affect my own power, which included my joy, happiness, peace, and love. I gave other people my power through being angry, upset, and unforgiving. *My unforgiveness and anger did not hurt anyone but me.* I had to accept some of the responsibility for what I was going through. I allowed and gave permission to the inconsiderate behavior and gave poor excuses for how others treated me. I decided to take ownership of my actions and the role that I played in my pain. Taking ownership of my actions by no means excuse any of the choices or behaviors that others may have made towards me during my grief recovery process. It simply allowed me to position myself to receive the freedom that I longed for and needed. I had to be honest in that I allowed myself to participate in unhealthy relationships and situations in my family and friend circles, and needed to change that. Because I failed to identify unhealthy relationships and set the proper boundaries in my life, my verbal and emotional response to each situation was not the best. The people who have hurt me whether they was family or friend, did not deserve my power. I was giving too much power to people who did not value my opinion, my existence, or how they treated me in the same way that I valued them. I discovered that each of us must come to terms with our flaws and take a healthy responsibility without diminishing our value. Most importantly, you can never have any peace, joy, or move forward in your recovery if you hold any resentment or anger towards other people, even if they hurt you during the grief and loss process of your mother. It is better to choose forgiveness than to harbor in resentment and to try to pay someone back that has hurt you that may not ever understand how he or she created your pain in the first place.

Making excuses for someone else who makes bad decisions empowers them to continue to make those same bad decisions. I began to do a self-evaluation of my life and friends after my mother passed away as I worked towards my healing. I had to ask myself some real questions. I mean, really get real about the relationships in my life: *"Are you getting poured into and are you pouring into them? Are you loving God and others more as a result of these relationships? Are you adding value to other people's lives? Are they adding value to you your life?"* just to name a few. If the answer was no, then I needed to distance myself from those relationships or seek to forgive them if I wanted to get out of my slump of pain from the loss of my mother. Therefore, making a better choice to embrace healthy relationships, remove the toxic relationships, and take the steps towards forgiveness was one of the best moves towards freedom that I could have ever made.

> *"Heal my wounds and broken heart. Please don't leave me in despair, in hurt, and in turmoil. Please don't leave me broken. I look forward to your mercy and love in my life. I will forgive and be an instrument used for the glory of the gospel."*
> ~ *Journal Entry*

Sense Of Responsibility

My mother gave birth to me at 21 years old. She was a young, married woman. Her skin and face were flawless. She always had a way of lighting up a room. She and I had been through a lot together. As mentioned, as the oldest, I would always watch my younger siblings, and I had a lot of responsibilities. I never minded though because I loved my family.

That structure may have caused a "sense of responsibility." So, I had a sense of responsibility to take care of my mom, to fight her battles, and to fix everything. I felt that her love and support were more than payment enough. Plus, I enjoyed it. It brought me great joy to bring her joy. However, just as it was unhealthy during her life, it became unhealthy when she passed away. I still carried that sense of responsibility with me even after she went home to be with the Lord.

Forgive Yourself

> *"I forgive myself for not being true to myself. I forgive myself for not allowing myself to be human. I forgive myself for not setting the right boundaries in the relationships in my life. I forgive myself for hurting others and making poor choices to hurt them back.*
> *I forgive myself for giving someone else my power."*
> *~ Journal Entry*

There is a purpose for our pain. We have to give ourselves permission to work through that pain discover our mission and purpose in life. We have to do it in a way that is healthy, and that is good. Sometimes we fall into the trap of blaming ourselves for something that was beyond our control. There may be times when we need to forgive ourselves for not allowing ourselves to be human. We have to forgive ourselves for carrying a burden that we were never meant to carry. So many people don't understand the fact that forgiving our own self is a part of our healing process. Losing a mother is hard. Whether you were a caregiver, or maybe not around, or whatever the case may be, you must forgive yourself. Holding on to pain in your heart against yourself will only hinder your life growth, not promote it. So decide today to forgive yourself. You can't hold on to burdens and pains in your heart for past mistakes or disagreements during the process of grief recovery.

Forgiving Others

It's tough for others to understand what it is like to be without your mom unless they have gone through it themselves or can empathize with another who has gone through the journey. At best they can empathize with the situation if they have an open mind and compassionate heart.

You may have to let go of the fact that some of the family or friends that are left behind, that you have selected to help you, may not provide you with the security, love, and support that you once had or believed that you had. It will be important to draw on your knowledge of who your mother was and attempt to live out the good that she wanted for you so that you can live a good and decent life. Most importantly, draw from who you are in Christ. Even if you did not have a good relationship with your mother, you can still live a better life than before, as a way to create a new path of healing for yourself.

The same rules apply for others. We may blame them and have anger towards them for something that we thought should have been done differently during our grief process. We may be angry with them if they did not help out as they should have, or if they did not help with the funeral, or if they were not there. There are so many things that we need to forgive others for. So in the same way, forgive them for their shortcomings and shortfalls. Not because they did not hurt you, but because you must live on in freedom for your dreams, goals, and more! Unforgiveness will only block your deliverance or ability to move on to true recovery after loosing a mother.

I know that these principles, though true, may seem a little out of the box. Forgiveness is the antidote the cures the deepest wounds in our hearts.

I had to learn to forgive others and allow them to live their own lives. We all have a life that we need to strive to live for. I finally decided to walk in my truth and allow for others to live in theirs. Holding on to things only made things worse. Forgiving others allows us to walk in love better and live better as people. I had to realize that my perspective is not the only way to view things. I had to accept that I was human, and so were those around me.

Our decision to look into the mirror at our own messy lives, make the decision to forgive, and process our journey in healthy way will determine how successful we will be in our recovery. The passing of my mother alone caused a lot of pain, but the events and the discovery of how relationships were around me made that season more intense. If I did not face those other moving pieces of my life, then it would not have been possible to recover or heal from loosing my mother. Little did I know that all of those moving pieces in my life were playing a role in my recovery and how I would heal from the pain of loss? In the same manner, you may have many moving pieces in your life that may determine how you will move on. It will be hard for you to get your true healing without forgiveness. Forgiveness is your secret ingredient and healing antidote. Forgive yourself and allow yourself to be human—especially when talking about our mother.

Freedom With Forgiveness
Making It Personal

Do you struggle with unforgiveness towards others surrounding the loss of your mother? Who are the people and what are the issues that have hurt you and why? Write it down. Look over your list. Make the decision today to forgive those who have hurt you so that you can move forward in your healing process.

"Dear Mommy, how are you? I miss you deeply. Things are horrible since you left. Well Mom, I have some things to get off my chest too. Mommy, you hurt me because of some of the decisions you made…What happened? You were my mom. You were supposed to protect me. Mom, you hurt me with your choices. I am angry because I felt that you abandoned me, betrayed me, and left me here alone. I am hurt in my soul. And I feel like you left me figure life out alone.
I felt like a part of me died with you.
But I can't go on like this. I want to be free and whole again.
Freedom is best. I choose to be free…
Mommy, I forgive you. I forgive you for the choices that you made concerning me. I forgive you for hurting me. I forgive you for not recognizing the signs of my pain better. I forgive you for falling short of protecting me.
I recognize you were a woman, mother, lover, and human. You were my mom. God is my God.

Therefore, I forgive you and release this forever."
~ Journal Entry

Forgiving Your Mother (even if she is not here)

It had been a long time since I had a vacation. I was longing for some time away. My husband and I wanted to celebrate our wedding anniversary. I thought it would be a great time to get away and enjoy the sun. Also, I had some things on my mind about my journey, and I thought a nice beach vacation would help me to process them. I made sure that I took my journal on this trip because I wanted to have it just in case I felt inspired to write. Up until that point, I had recognized many truths about my life and my mother. I needed to gain closure. The Riviera Maya seemed like the best place to start. It was where my husband and I had taken our first honeymoon, and we were now celebrating our eighth wedding anniversary.

It is said that the number eight represents new beginnings. I was looking forward to celebrating new beginnings in my marriage and possibly closure on my issues with my mother.

I could not wait to get to our all-inclusive resort so that I could enjoy the sun and beach. Plus, I was excited to have some reconnection time with my husband. We hadn't had a vacation together alone without the kids in years. Our lives had become so busy with work and the kids that we had failed to really date and connect with one another as we ought.

The Riviera Maya was amazing. The resort, food, and weather were great. The sunshine and warmth inspired happiness in my soul. It felt like a funny dream for us to be away without the kids. There wasn't anyone calling our names a hundred times or pampers to change or sippy cups to refill. Nor were there any calls from the office, meetings to attend, or presentations to prepare. It was just us. We needed this. We needed to connect with just us. Like we did originally. We had been through a lot when I had our children, endured life issues, took care of my sick mother, and then buried her. We almost didn't make it as a couple, and as a family. But God's grace was sufficient. We were able to get to the other side of the trauma stronger than ever. So, to enjoy this time away with my special man, my husband, my Boaz, my beloved, was everything.

In the midst of a storm, it may seem like a married couple cannot see the other side of the trial, but the joy and pleasure that a couple can have in their hearts when they get to the other side of a storm is priceless. The journey travelled together to acquire the testimony of victory after going through a tough trial, can cause a couple to have love and admiration for each other, in a much more meaningful and deeper way that is unselfish and unashamed. Both persons in a marriage come to the realization that they both have flaws, that there will be issues, and there may be things that will never change or be understood, but as a couple they can choose to submit to God and learn something different in order to leverage their best and most meaningful gifts and attributes to love each other and to promote the family union. That is what happened with us. So this trip was a symbol of forgiveness for each other, to start over in our relationship, have some fun time together, and to afford me the possibility of closure to leave my past in the past to heal from my grief.

Throughout my journey of grief, as I said before, I had placed my mother on a pedestal. I did not take a close look at her humanity and the decisions that she may have made that could have played a role in my frustration and dismay.

One of the most mature moments that I had was when I had to discover that my mother was human and may have not always made the decisions that I would have liked her to make, but she made decisions based upon what was in front of her at the time. All of the decisions that she made were not intended to hurt me or to spite me. One thing for sure was that she loved all of her children and did the best that she could. Her love was a great example for me as a mother, and a model that I try to share with my own children.

Even though her choices may not have been intentionally placed into motion to hurt me, I was still very angry with my mother and needed to forgive her. I blamed her for many things, especially when it came to her relationship with my father and how we had unresolved issues for so long. I blamed her for her role in the breakdown in the relationship between my father and I because she never addressed it openly. Though I loved her peacemaker capabilities, I was upset with how she did not engage completely into resolving the issues and took a more passive approach. Deep down inside, I think I wished that she had facilitated more conversation between us and noticed that I did want a relationship with my father, but we needed more help and my father needed to be accountable to being my father in other meaningful ways.

I viewed my mother's passive approach to my father and I relationship, as unhealthy. In a way, she did protect me, but she also protected him. She wanted to keep him in a good light and keep him active in my life. But she failed to realize, that he was already in a good light in my eyes. It was his lack of connection and empathy towards me that created the dark shadows of discord. Her way was not the best way. The way that she decided to handle things by taking my side sparked resentment and jealousy from others. The way she covered up for the issues in the background with my father caused hurt and pain. I was angry with my mother for not addressing it sooner and I was upset that I had to deal with it alone when she passed away.

My Mother As A Woman

I realized that my mother made the best decisions she could that would work for the life that she had. She was juggling between two people that she loved. I may not have liked her choices, but those were the ones that she made. I had to discover that my mother, just like others, was a *woman*. Mothers are regular human beings. They may seem like super-women in our eyes because they are our mothers, but they are working towards managing and living their lives just like anyone else. Though we may not agree with what they do, they are making choices in their lives about how they will handle the life that was dealt to them. They are also sisters, daughters, co-workers, and best friends—and since we are here, they were someone's love interest, significant other, wife, girlfriend, or lover. Our mothers have laughed, cried, cheered, and loved. They were in relationships with various people that turned them into who they were. They had experiences and decisions as grown women, and they lived their life as they chose to.

It is okay to disagree with your mother's decisions if the decisions she made may have hurt you. Forgiveness allows us to have freedom from their choices. This type of freedom allows us to accept the truth of who our mothers were to us and places us in position to receive our healing when they pass away. When a person who has lost a mother has not faced their truth and forgive, then they will go in an endless cycle of hurt and pain like a merry go round.

I owed it to myself to allow the hurt and pain from my mother go and to forgive her.

Therefore, I made the decision to let go of the things that I could not control and lay aside the questions that I will never receive an answer for. I made the decision to allow myself to heal, to forgive, and to live. I made the decision to extend to her the same grace, that if needed, that I would desire to receive.

Releasing My Forgiveness

After a nice beachfront dinner, I decided that it would be the perfect evening to go to the beach to write in my journal. I grabbed my journal, my favorite pen, and a glass of wine. I told my husband that I was going to the beach to spend some time with my journal and not to wait up. I walked to the beach and found an empty cabana. Beach was empty but very beautiful as the moon glistened over the ocean. I placed my belongings on the small table next to the lounge chair. I stretched out across the lounge chair and closed my eyes to experience the breeze across my face. The atmosphere was beautiful and peaceful. I felt inspired to write, as though the stage was set for such a moment as this. I took a sip from my glass of wine, opened my journal, and began to write. I wrote out all my thoughts on paper. I just let my heart flow, and my pen did not stop. I did not hold anything back. I was determined to get my freedom. I was in pursuit of moving forward. I was determined that even though she wasn't there, I wasn't going to be held hostage to unforgiveness towards her any longer.

I wrote *I forgive you.*

Ideally, I would have liked to have spoken with my mother face to face at a kitchen table or even in a counselor's office. I would have like to have been able to look her in her eyes and say what was on my mind and tell her exactly how I felt. In a perfect world, maybe I would have gotten an apology or perhaps she would have seen things my way. Yet, I learned in my healing process that when it comes to forgiveness, or in this case forgiving your mother, even if she is passed away, does not require for them to be present in order to forgive them or to get closure. We do not need to see them face-to-face or look them in the eyes in order to receive the promise of peace or to move forward. They do not need to apologize to us or see things our way. Our faith to forgive according to God's word is all we need to get closure. We can forgive by faith even if they are not there. Forgiveness is the key to closure. If we don't forgive and release that person whether they are living or not, we will replay in our minds over and over and over again the many conversations, issues, and problems that we may have faced. However, by forgiving our mothers, even if they are no longer living, we allow ourselves the opportunity to have complete closure and allow for the Holy Spirit to heal our hearts and to move forward in our new normal.

Grace To Forgive

If you are like me, who put your irreplaceable mother on an unhealthy pedestal of perfection, or who is angry that she has passed on, you are not alone. Now is the time to forgive and to release that anger against her. It may not happen overnight. It is okay if this takes some time. When you choose to forgive your mother, you receiving your recovery. The grace to forgive your mother is there even when she is not. You are the only person that is required to attend the forgiveness ceremony.

Decide today that you will make the decision to forgive your mother, even if she is not here. Be real about your thoughts and feelings. Allow your soul to release all of your thoughts and feelings so that you can move forward in your new normal in power and in peace.

Forgiving Your Mother
(even if she is not here)
Making It Personal

After reading the last chapter, what did you learn about forgiveness? Did you know that you could possibly have an issue with your mother that you need to address? Have you considered that you may have experienced hurt, pain, and turmoil in this season of grief because of the choices that were made by your mother? Are you willing to see her humanity and her flaws with love, and forgive them so that you may live a great life?

"I am writing this letter as a form of release of forgiveness and healing for me. The elders in my life have been wonderful in some areas but they also had caused much pain by not stepping in. I am humbled and thankful for all the good that they did, but I wished that they did not overlook the issues or turn the other way. I wanted to share my heart and forgive the elders in my life."

~ *Journal Entry*

Forgiving The Elder Figures

Forgiving My Grandparents

While I was on the beach, I also decided to write a letter to my grandfather. I was writing a letter to him because of the troubled relationship I was having with my father, and I had a longing for my grandfather to take more of an active role in the relationship between my father and I. My grandfather had already passed away at 90 years old a few years before my mother passed away. It seems as though there was a season of people who were passing away in our family back to back. My grandfather and I couldn't speak anymore, but I needed to get closure and forgive so that I can receive all the promises that God had for me. I did not want to leave any stone unturned.

My grandfather was the silent strong type. He was always a family man, strong individual, and hard worker. Hard work and a strong work ethic are character traits that run in my family. My grandfather was the ideal grandparent. He took us out to various places, watched us after school, attended our school events, and cooked some of the best meals during the holidays. As a grandfather, overall I did not have any complaints. My grandmother and I had a decent relationship but we would tend to have discord whenever there was discord with my father. I did have a concern that required me to forgive with regards to their silence about the breakdown in the relationship between my father and I, and at times the covering up of the issues. I felt as though they made a lot of excuses for him. If I had it my way, I would have liked to have the experience of accountability and forgiveness in my family, instead of excuses. When it came to my grandfather, I had to forgive him without him being present because he had already passed away. Ideally, I would have like to have met with my grandfather face to face, but wasn't case nor was it needed to accomplish the task. It would have been great to sit in a room together so that I could share with him my ideas and thoughts. When it came to my grandparents, I would have loved to share everything that I was thinking and the transformation that I had experience thus far. I wanted them to feel my pain and get clarity about my perspective about how I felt things were handled. Let's be honest. That type of conversation may not have changed much, and even if it did, the situations have already passed.

As I mentioned, face-to-face conversation is not necessary for forgiveness. As long as you and the Holy Spirit are present, you can forgive any person who has ever wronged or hurt you. Many times we get into the trap of thinking that we can only forgive if the person who hurt us is alive and that it is too late to forgive once they have died. Forgiveness doesn't have a timeline. It is not controlled by time. It is ready when you are ready. We have to remember that unforgiveness can hinder us from living the life that we desire to live or from reaching the place of healing that we desire after we lose our mother.

I wrote my letter to my grandfather, and grandmother. As I lay on the beach, I began to pour my heart out to my grandparents. I felt a sense of release as I put my thoughts and feelings on paper and let go of the unforgiveness against them. I shared my thoughts, and I expressed my forgiveness. I had every intention that I would live the best life I could. Not just for me, but for my family. I was committed to striving to live the best life I could.

I approached this part of the healing journey in part an example for my own children, so that they can see how to live on, forgive others, love your family, and move on to greater things no matter what obstacles that they may face. Closure comes from getting into agreement with Christ and acting on the Word of God to achieve the best results. If I were to pass away, I know I am going to heaven. I will be with Jesus. I will not hold any grudges against anyone. I will not be upset at the last things that people said or did not say. I would not even care. I would want them to live on while giving consideration and support to those around them that are grieving. I forgave for myself, but I also forgave so that my children, grand-children, and great-grand children could have an example of how to offer forgiveness and live out their full potential if they were to able come across hard times in their life.

Forgiving My Father

> *"Lord, I just want my heart to dance. I want my heart to be overjoyed and active. Lord, I forgive my father. I forgive him for everything. I let it go. From the woman, I am today, to the hurt little girl on the inside of me that doesn't understand why my dad can't love me.. I let it all go. I forgive my father."*
>
> *~ Journal Entry*

Years had passed since I had been to the Riviera Maya. I was going about my life, and I was focused on raising a family and working. Then, I started to deal with the issue of my father. He and I had a broken relationship. I believed that I had moved on from our issues, so I was surprised when I started to think about him again.

As I have shared, our relationship has always been a trouble point for me, especially as a believer. On one hand, I would go to church and learn about God, and about how forgiving, loving, and kind He was. But on the other hand, my relationship with my biological father needed repair and restoration.

One weekend, I went to on a retreat to unravel my thoughts and to get some time away to myself. I had been so focused on taking care of the family that I took some time for myself. I had plans to just release my nagging frustrations and to move forward. I opened up one of my journals and began to read about my heartache and pain from the relationship with my father. I wrote the entries as they occurred, but I had not read them in years. I read my words about the things that had been done and said to me over the years. I remembered the pain and the betrayal that I had felt regarding them. As I reminisced over those times, I began to weep. I mean really weep about my experiences. I had not cried liked that over any major situation in a long time.

I realized in that moment that I had never really wept over my pain or the pain that I had regarding my father. I had just moved on like nothing had happened. I buried the issue and continued to move forward. I was lying in my bed, holding my journal, and weeping like a baby. I was a mature woman at the time, but the person crying in that hotel room was the little girl on the inside of me who did not understand why her daddy did not love her as she needed. I had not realized that I needed to deal with the pain. I had not even realized that it was an issue. The emotional and spiritual disconnect was extremely painful for me as it left me feeling invisible and invalidated for many years and with many people.

For years, I thought I had it under control and was okay. Yet, I discovered in that moment, that I needed to forgive my father. My eyes were red and full of tears as I prayed a prayer to forgive my father. I said, "*I forgive my father.*"

As I was crying and began to experience relief, I sensed a small voice in heart that said, "*Now you can write your book.*"

I was in awe and so surprised! I had attempting to write this book for a while and had not been able to finish. However, all of this time, the reason that I had not finished writing this book was because I was missing a key ingredient. I could not finish writing it until I had forgiven my father. The last piece to this book was *forgiveness*.

I had to forgive my father and let go of the past and pain.

I did know that the forgiveness of my father, my known rival, was the last piece of the puzzle. My concerns that I had with my father were also connected to the issues I had with my mother and was blocking my grief recovery. I cried that night because of the pain from the relationship but also because of the relief. I felt like there was a weight was lifted off my shoulders.

Forgiving my father, who was still alive, did not mean that I could just act as if nothing had happened or simply welcome him into my life at every angle. What it did mean was that I was able to acknowledge that I was not happy with some of his choices, and with discretion could make my own choices as to how and what kind of relationship I wanted to have with him according to how I chose.

The relationship with my father created many wonderful learning experiences and opportunities that I will be forever grateful for. For one, I was able to experience the security of a father figure by having a father present in my life. My father taught me valuable lessons about life, business, and men that helped me navigate through the waters of the world, and without that, I may have been very lost. I will always be grateful for those things. On the other side, because of our emotional and spiritual disconnect, the relationship left me with a void that allowed me to feel and understand the sense of what it means to not have a father. Therefore, God used my situation to develop the ability to speak to multiple people and connect to them in a real way. I can speak to people who have had a good connection with their father in their lives and relate to the joyful experiences that that type of relationship would bring. He also made it possible for me to connect with people who have not had a father and to connect to their pain as well. The Lord gave me a desire to learn and to seek truth, and used it in the midst of my brokenness to find the truth in His word on how to handle to real-world situations including how to heal after a mother passes away from an illness such as cancer. I believe that the Lord had a greater plan for the discord and disconnect between my father and I that will help many others in their journey. God knew I would one day discover to find the best answers I could to receive my healing. My mother was my best friend, and I could not continue in the pain of her loss forever. I believe that there were many others like me that He wanted me to reach. It was not just for me or about me. It was for someone else that He wanted to reach, touch, and help in the world.

We all have some sort of complicated relationship. Many of us may have a similar story. Perhaps we have a father figure who we are not close to, but we need to forgive. Our forgiveness does not mean that we approve or condone their poor choices; nor does it give them a free pass to the next birthday party. However, it does release our hearts and minds from the bondage of unforgiveness and anger. If the relationship and healing is salvageable and reconciliation is possible, then that is great, but if the relationship is too toxic, then it may be best to exercise prudence in maintaining a healthy distance to remain focused on the decision to forgive and walk in love. Some choices are best executed from afar if necessary.

My Father As A Man

I had to learn my father's story too. I had to understand that he is also a human being just like I am. He was a boy who turned into a man very early in life and did the best he could do with the hand he was dealt. My father instilled hard work into each of us and expected us to excel in everything that we did. He too has had his own struggles, loss, pain, betrayals, trials, and tribulations. He was no more of superman that I was a superwoman. I could not place him only in the dog house, no more than I could place my mother only on a pedestal as if she did not have a role to play. He made choices that I did not agree with, but so does anyone else. There came a point to where I had to decide if I was going to live on in my new normal in forgiveness that I had to let go of harboring the pain of our relationship. If I was going to life the life full of freedom and peace that I had to acknowledge that he had a story too. My father has accomplished more in his life than most men could ever say or do, not only through his own success but through the accomplishments of his children, as mostly all of us finished college, have technical trades, or successful businesses. I personally think that was why it was hard to get through to him about the need to make certain adjustments because he had tunnel vision about success for his kids and family. Everything else was secondary. The fact that his children were able to have more and do more was satisfactory for him, and according to his personality.

Not forgetting that he loved my mother. She was the wife of his youth. My mother was his ride or die, his best friend, and confidant. I am sure that the friendship that they had played a role as to why he supported her through the chemo process. He had a relationship with my mother. In our family dynamic, she had certain responsibilities and he had his. In his own journey, he may have felt lost, scared, or confused on how to manage his children without her. There were certain responsibilities and family activities that he did not have to worry about when my mother was alive because it was considered 'her thing'. However, after she passed away those things became responsibilities for him. Even though our disconnection had a lot of history, I am confident that he had to adjust to being without my mother as well.

In my life, most of my entrepreneurial go get 'em attitude, and work ethic come from my father. My family and academia drive came from both of my parents. My father pushed me hard, but it was also that push that helped me to succeed. Therefore, I decided that holding onto the unforgiveness towards my father, even if our exchanges were harsh and hurtful, wasn't going to hurt him or even make him "get it." It wasn't necessary for he and I to have to same opinions about life in order for me to forgive him and live in freedom. I simply needed to get into agreement with the Word of God, trust God, and take action by faith to mature as a believer. In other words, I needed to forgive!

Do you have a similar story? Can you relate to the complexity of forgiveness with a surviving parent? As I shared, your story my have similar qualities but just a different twist depending on the characters and the plot. We all have our own path to take. My father, along with those in your life that have you have complex relationships with, will experience the same loving kindness at the end of their journey as you will. I too will need God's grace and mercy in my own life and choices. I will not be the perfect parent. There are not any play books to parenting. Understand, that my forgiveness of my father or any person does not excuse their behavior, actions, or even place them in a close relationship with me. Forgiveness does not grant a person a ticket into our lives or access into our happiness. It simply means that our Father will look at my father and your father-figure or any person with love, compassion, and understanding according to His will. It was not easy. But I decided that forgiveness was the best thing to do, for me. I did not need him to be present for me to forgive. I did not need him to agree with me to forgive. I did not need him to understand or connect with me to forgive. I had my own agreement, my own prayers, and my own commitment with my Heavenly Father and the Word of God to live free, and that was all I needed.

Forgiving the Father or Father Figure in your life

Forgiving a father or father figure is not about them, but about you. We were not there when they grew up; we don't know what experiences they had or the effects of those experiences on their lives. We do not forgive our fathers or father figures to give them excuses, but to give us freedom. Their choices do not determine our value. I encourage you, if applicable to your situation, to choose forgiveness for yourself and release the issues that you may have with the father or father figure in your life.

Forgiving The Father Figures
Making It Personal

Have you experienced hurt, pain, or disappointment from your father or father figure? Are you in a place where you can forgive even if you don't have a relationship with him? Realizing that our fathers are just as human as our mothers and that they too can make mistakes, how can we move forward without allowing their choices to hinder our growth?

Acceptance For "The New Normal"

"Father, I thank you for this new season. I feel hope again. I may not like what has happened, but I am finally at a point where I can accept it. I am no longer afraid of it. I have a future ahead of children and me that need me. I know that I can make it as long as I have you. The future looks bright and I am excited about what is to come."

~ *Journal Entry*

Acceptance

When coming to a place of acceptance, there is liberation and freedom because you know that life will move on. You may not know how all things will happen, but it will work in your favor. Acceptance is the ultimate goal to grief recovery but at times is a difficult thing. It is hard to grasp the pain of losing a mother who you care so much about and you may not want to accept the reality that it has happened. This is true even if you did not have the best relationship with your mother figure. At times, we may not even realize that we do not want to accept it. I know that in my case I was afraid of what was on the other side. To move into acceptance would have meant that I needed to admit that my mother was gone. To accept that she was gone was almost unimaginable. To accept that I would have to continue on this journey without my irreplaceable mother was not something I was looking forward to. But I had gotten to a place in my life where I was so tired of being tired. I was tired of not living out my full potential and purpose as a woman, wife, and mother. I wanted to live out my life in front of my children in a way that would show them my faith, life, joy, and what was taught to me by mother. I wanted to show my kids who my mother was through our relationship and through stories. My mother was a happy and joyful woman, so I needed to get to a place where my life reflected that to them.

Allowing myself to be liberated from the past, forgiving others, and releasing the negativity and opinions of others, was the best decision I could have made, and the best one you can make too. I didn't need to be overtaken by negative thoughts and emotions. I decided to smile, to live, and experience love by letting down the walls that I had built up in my life after my mother passed away but it was time to take them down. Love is a beautiful thing because it can be experienced. Even if at times it breaks our hearts or doesn't turn out, as we would like, we should never regret loving any person especially not our mothers.

Perhaps there has been a wall up during your grief process that has kept relationships from growing or blossoming that now in this phase of your life you could entertain rebuilding. Nonetheless, allowing the walls to come down and the healing to flow lets us experience the recovery that we desire. Step into the season of acceptance so that you can experience the complete recovery that you desire.

Hope

I am not done with this journey of self-discovery after losing my mother. I have not arrived. I am on the journey with you. Know that this is a journey, not a destination. Your mother will always be with you. She is a part of you. If you spend a lot of time trying to get rid of her, you may begin to feel stuck again. We have hope that we will continue to make it and be more than overcomers in the world. We will live a life that is victorious. This is a promise to us.

> *"...in all these things we are more than conquerors through him who loved us."*
> *Romans 8:37*

It is like having a prosthetic leg. You have a new leg, and it works, but it's not like the original. You are happy, but it is new. So losing your mother is like trying to get by with the prosthetic leg. If you want to cry—cry. If you want to yell—yell. Don't be afraid to be yourself. Live for yourself and be sure to continue to look up. It only gets better from here. Day by day, week-by-week, and year-by-year, you will discover how to get through the adjustment to life without your mom. It is not about acting as though losing her did not have any effect on you. It is about recognizing that it did, and you are using that pain to make you stronger, to make you better.

You will overcome this. This will be one of the best learning experiences that you have ever had. You may discover a greater purpose for your pain and loss. Look at me, I am here writing a book on a subject that I did not think I would or could write, but look at what God decided to do. So, as you go through this journey don't dismiss the possibility of reaching into a new normal that is grand, beautiful and new.

Have hope for a better future. You will have strength as you continue forth in your journey with hope, power, and purpose.

Be Yourself

The best advice I ever received when I started my walk in Christ was to be myself. I'll share that same advice with you once again. Each of us are unique and have a plan for our lives. Some people will always want to put you in a box. Don't do it. Jump out of it or carve arms out of it if you need to in order to make it your own.

When I recognized my need to accept my mother's passing, I prayed this prayer:

"Father, give me guidance, wisdom, and strength to accept the passing of my mother. Please help me stay the course of the decisions that I have made to forgive, remove myths, and to live a healthy life since my mother has passed away. I declare that I accept by faith that my mother has passed away and I will live a new normal life with joy, peace, and healing in my heart. In Jesus Name."

Acceptance
Making It Personal

Acceptance is an important step in the journey. What could you do to accept the passing of your mother? Now that you have forgiven others who have hurt you, can you accept that healing to move into your new normal?

The "New Normal"

The "New Normal" is your new, normal way of life after your irreplaceable mother has passed away. I was skeptical about moving forward because I was afraid but God showed me that it was possible. Sometimes when we may feel like there is a lot of pain from losing an irreplaceable mother, we tend to stay away from accepting the new normal. Starting to understand and accept that death is a part of life means that we can begin to look forward again. For those who have faith in Christ, that death is not the end of life, but the beginning of a better, eternal life in heaven with Jesus Christ.

We do not need to fear our new normal but to embrace it! Our new normal is filled with new memories, new traditions, and a new way of life. Most importantly, our new normal is a demonstration of our transformation.

Our Heavenly Father is aware of how we valued our irreplaceable mother. That is why it is so amazing to think about how one day there will no longer be any death, and we will be reunited with our loved one. Yet, in the meantime, we will continue in joy as individuals who trust God.

When we decide to live out our new normal, it does not mean that we do not feel any emotions or no longer have any trials. It simply means that we are moving toward our joy each day by faith. We decided lean forward and to bend our hearts forward in Him.

Our mothers may be gone, but we are here to live on in power, freedom, and healing. Some of us are parents, may one day become parents, or know what it is like to see someone else's child in pain. We must ask ourselves how we would want to have our children live on. I know that for me, I want my children to live on and have happy healthy live in their power, with joy, in unity with each other, and with strong faith in Christ. My children will not ever have to worry about where I am after my home going. They can have confidence that their mother is a Believer and is home with Jesus. My prayer is that I will develop to be their irreplaceable mother. I am grateful for them, for they gave me a reason to live, to strive, and move forward. They inspired my hopes and dreams and kept me on the right path. In the same way, many times our mothers do the best they can, but in the end, we have to move forward to live the life we were destined to live.

Some people may not feel that they are ready to move forward into their new normal without their mother, but it is the final step that is necessary for the complete healing. It is difficult, trying to move on and accept the fact that our mother is no longer there. Be sure to open your heart to new things.

We become the new matriarchs or the new leaders. Sometimes we become the heads of our families. When you lose a mother, you have dual roles of functioning both within your generation and within the one that she left behind. Be real with yourself and walk in your truth.

I don't think I will ever be completely okay with the fact that my mother is gone. I would give anything just to spend some time with her again. But in the same manner, I don't think I would have grown in the way I have as a Believer, woman, wife, daughter, sister, aunt, friend, and mother if I had not experienced the pain of losing her. The pain of her passing brought a level of brokenness and heartbreak that opened my soul to discover some truths about my life and myself. My faith in God is deeper. My love for my family is stronger. My sense of value is greater and more purposeful. I live each day with purpose, thinking of my children. Thinking of the legacy that I will leave to them. I want them to live their best life for their entire life. I would always want them to rejoice in Christ, whether I am with them or with the Lord, knowing that as their mother I found my new normal after losing my mother, and in their season if they lose me, that they too will find their new normal, in Christ, and with focus and love for each other and for their future.

I want to say, congratulations on investing in your and receiving your recovery, restoration, and healing. Your future is bright! It only gets better from here.

To God be the glory for always for our journeys, testimonies, and growth. I love you, Father! I love you, Jesus Christ! Thank you for the journey! That you for letting me be real and never letting me go!

I am rooting for you. You can do this. This is something that you will overcome and learn from. You have a great purpose in your life. I pray that in your journey of healing after loosing your Irreplaceable Mother, that you will find freedom, balance, and faith for your victory.

The New Normal
Making It Personal

What can you do to begin your new lease on life in your new normal? What kind of activities will you begin today? What are you looking forward to with your new normal?

APPENDIX

What If My Mother Passed Away While I Was Young?

If your mother passed away while you were young, then you can have closure. Never limit your deliverance based upon time and material things. Your deliverance is based upon what you do and have right now. Gather as much information as you possibly can and try to be the best you can be for your healing from grief.

There is never a good age to lose a parent, but if it happens when we are young, we can feel as though our lives could have been better if they were still here. Or feel as though we were cheated out of having that relationship. There is no denying that losing a parent at a young age is a difficult truth to take on, but it is not a truth that gives you automatic permission to remain stuck. A person who loses their mother at a young age will still need to grieve and mourn, if it is not for anything other than to grieve and mourn what they did not experience.

The only person who is required to be present for your deliverance and healing is you. No one else is required to be in attendance. So, if your mother passed away while you were young, then that means you would have to go through life without having her there physically. But, she is there with you in spirit and heart. God is with you. You are never alone. A mother desires for her child to move on and to trust in the process, even if it does not make sense. It is okay to miss her or to long for her. That is normal. I am not aware of an expiration date of how long you can miss your mother, so feel free to always miss her. Yet, your decision to miss her should not allow you to hinder your growth and success in the long run. Remember, God is in control. We may not have all of the answers, but we have to trust the process of life. Your mother passing away when you are young has nothing to do with your self-worth or value as much as it had to do with life and the fact that it was her time to go home to be with the Lord. So, live your life knowing that God is sovereign. There is never a good age to lose a mother. So no matter how old you were, you will be fine.

The Journey Into Adulthood

When a young person loses a mother, they have to take the journey into adulthood without the physical guidance of that parent. In those cases, it is important to find out as much as you can about that person, so that you can discover more about them to help you lead your own life. It can also help to find mentors and other women who can step in and discuss issues and life with you. You can never have too much support. The most important thing is to know that the heart of a mother is for her babies to move on and live great lives. You do this by living the life you need to live and being victorious in your life.

What If I Had A Poor Relationship With My Mother?

Not every relationship we have is one that we desire. We would love to believe that each person had this relationship with his or her mother where they were best friends, but the truth of it is that some relationships may not have blossomed as we hoped. One thing we need to discover is that our healing is not based upon whether or not we have a good relationship with the other party or not.

Many times we run into obstacles when there is a mother figure that is not nurturing or able to give love, as we would like to receive it. We have to remember that we are not responsible for whether or not they were able to love us in the fashion that we desired. We may never know or understand the reasons for what they do. The only thing that we can be responsible for is making sure that whatever we do in our current situation and our future is a reflection of the healthy and happy life we desire.

So, even if your relationship with your mother was not the best, does not mean that you may not experience grief about her passing. You may still experience the stages of grief and have all of the same experiences. Therefore, you should still go through the journey of recovery. The poor relationship with your mother also does not mean that you are to be trapped by guilt and despair because things were not rosy between you. She was an adult. You are or will be an adult yourself. You cannot be responsible for her actions. You can only be responsible for yours.

Therefore, decide today to have your recovery and your freedom.

Dealing with the Hand That Was Dealt

Imagine a deck of cards. You just shuffle and get the cards that are dealt. In life, there are things that we are handed that are out of our control. We have to roll with the punches. Therefore, we can only respond to what we have. So, if you did not have the relationship you desired that is okay because you can still receive healing from your pain.

Encouragement For The Holidays

The holiday season is a popular and busy time of year. In our home, it is filled with faith reflections, family traditions, thanksgiving, and family activities. The majority of my upbringing was filled with family traditions and activities, and now I plan such things for my own family.

If you are struggling through the holiday season, you are not alone. This is the time to create new traditions and to find a way to symbolize that person's life so that you can live on and prosper. Things may not be the same, but it is not necessary for them to be so because this is our new normal.

New Traditions

During this process, it is hard to go through the holidays as before. It is not uncommon that the holidays become times that are not filled with joy. Use this time to find your own voice and ground to love and build your own life, and perhaps your family, to the glory of God.

Salvation (Sinners') Prayer

If you desire to have a relationship with God and Father that I spoke about in this book, I want to congratulate you on making an amazing decision! To accept Christ into you life, and start a relationship with our Heavenly Father starts with the prayer below. Please pray the below prayer. Once you have completed this prayer, I encourage you to find a good local church to get connected to so that you can start the path of learning more about your faith.

"Dear Father in Heaven, I come to You in the name of Jesus. I acknowledge to You that I am a sinner, and I repent for my sins and the life that I have lived; I need your forgiveness.
I believe that You are the only begotten Son Jesus Christ that shed His precious blood on the cross at Calvary and died
You said in Your word, Romans 10:9, that if we confess the Lord our God and believe in our hearts that God raised Jesus from the dead, we shall be saved.
Right now I confess Jesus as the Lord of my soul. With my heart, I believe that God raised Jesus from the dead. This very moment I accept Jesus Christ as my own personal Savior, and according to His Word, right now I am saved.
Thank you Father that I am now saved, forgiven, and adopted into your family!
In Jesus name,
Amen"

If you prayed the above prayer, and would like to get some additional resources to help you on your journey, please email us at theirreplaceablemother@gmail.com and put in the subject line: "New Friend".

Scriptures For Comfort

In times of grief recovery, it can be very helpful to create confessions and prayer. I have found these scriptures to be very comforting in my time of bereavement. I hope that they will help you to draw closer to God in your journey as well.

NUMBERS 6:24-26

"'The LORD bless you and keep you; the LORD make his face shine on you and be gracious to you; the LORD turn his face toward you and give you peace.'"

DEUTERONOMY 7:9

Know therefore that the LORD your God is God; he is the faithful God, keeping his covenant of love to a thousand generations of those who love him and keep his commandments.

JOB 19:25-27

I know that my redeemer lives, and that in the end he will stand on the earth. And after my skin has been destroyed, yet in my flesh I will see God; I myself will see him with my own eyes—I, and not another. How my heart yearns within me!

PSALM 18:4-6

The cords of death entangled me; the torrents of destruction overwhelmed me. The cords of the grave coiled around me; the snares of death confronted me. In my distress I called to the LORD; I cried to my God for help. From his temple he heard my voice; my cry came before him, into his ears.

PSALM 18:16-19

He reached down from on high and took hold of me; he drew me out of deep waters. He rescued me from my powerful enemy, from my foes, who were too strong for me. They confronted me in the day of my disaster, but the LORD was my support. He brought me out into a spacious place; he rescued me because he delighted in me.

PSALM 23:1-3

The LORD is my shepherd, I lack nothing. He makes me lie down in green pastures, he leads me beside quiet waters, he refreshes my soul. He guides me along the right paths for his name's sake.

PSALM 27:13-14

I remain confident of this: I will see the goodness of the LORD in the land of the living. Wait for the LORD; be strong and take heart and wait for the LORD.

PSALM 30:5

For his anger lasts only a moment, but his favor lasts a lifetime; weeping may stay for the night, but rejoicing comes in the morning.

PSALM 30:10-12

"…Hear, LORD, and be merciful to me; LORD, be my help." You turned my wailing into dancing; you removed my sackcloth and clothed me with joy, that my heart may sing your praises and not be silent. LORD my God, I will praise you forever.

PSALM 31:24

Be strong and take heart, all you who hope in the LORD.

PSALM 32:7

You are my hiding place; you will protect me from trouble and surround me with songs of deliverance.

PSALM 34:17-19

The righteous cry out, and the LORD hears them; he delivers them from all their troubles. The LORD is close to the brokenhearted and saves those who are crushed in spirit. The righteous person may have many troubles, but the LORD delivers him from them all…

PSALM 42:1-3

As the deer pants for streams of water, so my soul pants for you, my God. My soul thirsts for God, for the living God. When can I go and meet with

God? My tears have been my food day and night, while people say to me all day long, "Where is your God?"

PSALM 42:5

Why, my soul, are you downcast? Why so disturbed within me? Put your hope in God, for I will yet praise him, my Savior and my God.

PSALM 46:1-2

God is our refuge and strength, an ever-present help in trouble. Therefore we will not fear, though the earth give way and the mountains fall into the heart of the sea...

PSALM 56:8-10

Record my misery; list my tears on your scroll—are they not in your record? Then my enemies will turn back when I call for help. By this I will know that God is for me. In God, whose word I praise, in the LORD, whose word I praise...

PSALM 61:1-4

Hear my cry, O God; listen to my prayer. From the ends of the earth I call to you, I call as my heart grows faint; lead me to the rock that is higher than I. For you have been my refuge, a strong tower against the foe. I long to dwell in your tent forever and take refuge in the shelter of your wings.

PSALM 92:1-2

It is good to praise the LORD and make music to your name, O Most High, proclaiming your love in the morning and your faithfulness at night...

PSALM 94:17-19

Unless the LORD had given me help, I would soon have dwelt in the silence of death. When I said, "My foot is slipping," your unfailing love, LORD, supported me. When anxiety was great within me, your consolation brought me joy.

PSALM 115:3

Our God is in heaven; he does whatever pleases him.

PSALM 139:13-14

For you created my inmost being; you knit me together in my mother's womb. I praise you because I am fearfully and wonderfully made; your works are wonderful, I know that full well.

PROVERBS 3:5-6

Trust in the LORD with all your heart and lean not on your own understanding; in all your ways submit to him, and he will make your paths straight.

PROVERBS 14:32

When calamity comes, the wicked are brought down, but even in death the righteous seek refuge in God.

PROVERBS 18:10

The name of the LORD is a fortified tower; the righteous run to it and are safe.

PROVERBS 29:18 (ASV)

Where there is no vision, the people cast off restraint; But he that keepeth the law, happy is he.

ISAIAH 40:11

He tends his flock like a shepherd: He gathers the lambs in his arms and carries them close to his heart; he gently leads those that have young.

ISAIAH 40:28

Do you not know? Have you not heard? The LORD is the everlasting God, the Creator of the ends of the earth. He will not grow tired or weary, and his understanding no one can fathom.

ISAIAH 57:1-2

The righteous perish, and no one takes it to heart; the devout are taken away, and no one understands that the righteous are taken away to be spared from evil. Those who walk uprightly enter into peace; they find rest as they lie in death.

ISAIAH 60:20

Your sun will never set again, and your moon will wane no more; the LORD will be your everlasting light, and your days of sorrow will end.

ISAIAH 61:1-3

The Spirit of the Sovereign LORD is on me, because the LORD has anointed me to proclaim good news to the poor. He has sent me to bind up the brokayenhearted, to proclaim freedom for the captives and release from darkness for the prisoners, to proclaim the year of the LORD's favor and the day of vengeance of our God, to comfort all who mourn, and provide for those who grieve in Zion—to bestow on them a crown of beauty instead of ashes, the oil of joy instead of mourning, and a garment of praise instead of a spirit of despair. They will be called oaks of righteousness, a planting of the LORD for the display of his splendor.

JEREMIAH 17:7-8

"But blessed is the one who trusts in the LORD, whose confidence is in him. They will be like a tree planted by the water that sends out its roots by the stream. It does not fear when heat comes; its leaves are always green. It has no worries in a year of drought and never fails to bear fruit."

JEREMIAH 29:11

"…For I know the plans I have for you," declares the LORD, "plans to prosper you and not to harm you, plans to give you hope and a future…"

JEREMIAH 29:13

You will seek me and find me when you seek me with all your heart.

LAMENTATIONS 3:22-24

Because of the LORD's great love we are not consumed, for his compassions never fail. They are new every morning; great is your faithfulness. I say to myself, "The LORD is my portion; therefore I will wait for him."

MATTHEW 5:4

Blessed are those who mourn, for they will be comforted.

MATTHEW 11:28-30

"Come to me, all you who are weary and burdened, and I will give you rest. Take my yoke upon you and learn from me, for I am gentle and humble in heart, and you will find rest for your souls. For my yokaye is easy and my burden is light."

JOHN 1:12

Yet to all who did receive him, to those who believed in his name, he gave the right to become children of God…

JOHN 12:24

Very truly I tell you, unless a kernel of wheat falls to the ground and dies, it remains only a single seed. But if it dies, it produces many seeds.

JOHN 14:1-3

"Do not let your hearts be troubled. You believe in God; believe also in me. My Father's house has many rooms; if that were not so, would I have told you that I am going there to prepare a place for you? And if I go and prepare a place for you, I will come back and take you to be with me that you also may be where I am…"

JOHN 14:6

Jesus answered, "I am the way and the truth and the life. No one comes to the Father except through me…"

JOHN 14:16-18 (ASV)

And I will pray the Father, and he shall give you another Comforter, that he may be with you for ever, even the Spirit of truth: whom the world cannot receive; for it beholdeth him not, neither knoweth him: ye know him; for he abideth with you, and shall be in you. I will not leave you desolate: I come unto you.

JOHN 14:27-28

"…Peace I leave with you; my peace I give you. I do not give to you as the world gives. Do not let your hearts be troubled and do not be afraid.

"You heard me say, 'I am going away and I am coming back to you.' If you loved me, you would be glad that I am going to the Father, for the Father is greater than I…"

ROMANS 8:16

The Spirit himself testifies with our spirit that we are God's children.

ROMANS 8:23

Not only so, but we ourselves, who have the firstfruits of the Spirit, groan inwardly as we wait eagerly for our adoption to sonship, the redemption of our bodies.

ROMANS 8:28

And we know that in all things God works for the good of those who love him, who have been called according to his purpose.

ROMANS 8:31-32

What, then, shall we say in response to these things? If God is for us, who can be against us? He who did not spare his own Son, but gave him up for us all—how will he not also, along with him, graciously give us all things?

ROMANS 8:37-39

No, in all these things we are more than conquerors through him who loved us. For I am convinced that neither death nor life, neither angels nor demons, neither the present nor the future, nor any powers, neither height nor depth, nor anything else in all creation, will be able to separate us from the love of God that is in Christ Jesus our Lord.

ROMANS 12:2

Do not conform to the pattern of this world, but be transformed by the renewing of your mind. Then you will be able to test and approve what God's will is—his good, pleasing and perfect will.

ROMANS 15:4

For everything that was written in the past was written to teach us, so that through the endurance taught in the Scriptures and the encouragement they provide we might have hope.

ROMANS 15:13

May the God of hope fill you with all joy and peace as you trust in him, so that you may overflow with hope by the power of the Holy Spirit.

1 CORINTHIANS 15:25-26

For he must reign until he has put all his enemies under his feet. The last enemy to be destroyed is death.

1 CORINTHIANS 15:55

"Where, O death, is your victory? Where, O death, is your sting?"

2 CORINTHIANS 1:3-4

Praise be to the God and Father of our Lord Jesus Christ, the Father of compassion and the God of all comfort, who comforts us in all our troubles, so that we can comfort those in any trouble with the comfort we ourselves receive from God.

2 CORINTHIANS 5:1-4

For we know that if the earthly tent we live in is destroyed, we have a building from God, an eternal house in heaven, not built by human hands. Meanwhile we groan, longing to be clothed instead with our heavenly dwelling, because when we are clothed, we will not be found naked. For while we are in this tent, we groan and are burdened, because we do not wish to be unclothed but to be clothed instead with our heavenly dwelling, so that what is mortal may be swallowed up by life.

2 CORINTHIANS 12:9

But he said to me, "My grace is sufficient for you, for my power is made perfect in weakness." Therefore I will boast all the more gladly about my weaknesses, so that Christ's power may rest on me.

EPHESIANS 1:5

…he[a] predestined us for adoption to sonship through Jesus Christ, in accordance with his pleasure and will…

EPHESIANS 5:31-32

"For this reason a man will leave his father and mother and be united to his wife, and the two will become one flesh." This is a profound mystery—but I am talking about Christ and the church.

PHILIPPIANS 1:20

I eagerly expect and hope that I will in no way be ashamed, but will have sufficient courage so that now as always Christ will be exalted in my body, whether by life or by death.

PHILIPPIANS 3:20-21

But our citizenship is in heaven. And we eagerly await a Savior from there, the Lord Jesus Christ, who, by the power that enables him to bring everything under his control, will transform our lowly bodies so that they will be like his glorious body.

PHILIPPIANS 4:4

Rejoice in the Lord always. I will say it again: Rejoice!

PHILIPPIANS 4:6-9

Do not be anxious about anything, but in every situation, by prayer and petition, with thanksgiving, present your requests to God. And the peace of God, which transcends all understanding, will guard your hearts and your minds in Christ Jesus.

Finally, brothers and sisters, whatever is true, whatever is noble, whatever is right, whatever is pure, whatever is lovely, whatever is admirable—if anything is excellent or praiseworthy—think about such things. Whatever you have learned or received or heard from me, or seen in me—put it into practice. And the God of peace will be with you.

1 THESSALONIANS 4:13-18

Brothers and sisters, we do not want you to be uninformed about those who sleep in death, so that you do not grieve like the rest of mankind, who have no hope. For we believe that Jesus died and rose again, and so we believe that God will bring with Jesus those who have fallen asleep in him. According to the Lord's word, we tell you that we who are still alive, who are left until the coming of the Lord, will certainly not precede those who have fallen asleep. For the Lord himself will come down from heaven, with a loud command, with the voice of the archangel and with the trumpet call of God, and the dead in Christ will rise first. After that, we who are still alive and are left will be caught up together with them in the clouds to meet the Lord in the air. And so we will be with the Lord forever. Therefore encourage one another with these words.

1 THESSALONIANS 5:8-10

But since we belong to the day, let us be sober, putting on faith and love as a breastplate, and the hope of salvation as a helmet. For God did not appoint us to suffer wrath but to receive salvation through our Lord Jesus Christ. He died for us so that, whether we are awake or asleep, we may live together with him.

2 THESSALONIANS 2:16-17

May our Lord Jesus Christ himself and God our Father, who loved us and by his grace gave us eternal encouragement and good hope, encourage your hearts and strengthen you in every good deed and word.

2 TIMOTHY 1:12

That is why I am suffering as I am. Yet this is no cause for shame, because I know whom I have believed, and am convinced that he is able to guard what I have entrusted to him until that day.

2 TIMOTHY 4:7-8

I have fought the good fight, I have finished the race, I have kept the faith. Now there is in store for me the crown of righteousness, which the Lord, the righteous Judge, will award to me on that day—and not only to me, but also to all who have longed for his appearing.

TITUS 1:2

…in the hope of eternal life, which God, who does not lie, promised before the beginning of time…

TITUS 2:13

…while we wait for the blessed hope—the appearing of the glory of our great God and Savior, Jesus Christ…

HEBREWS 4:14-16

Therefore, since we have a great high priest who has ascended into heaven, Jesus the Son of God, let us hold firmly to the faith we profess. For we do not have a high priest who is unable to empathize with our weaknesses, but we have one who has been tempted in every way, just as we are—yet he did not sin. Let us then approach God's throne of grace with confidence, so that we may receive mercy and find grace to help us in our time of need.

HEBREWS 11:13-16

All these people were still living by faith when they died. They did not receive the things promised; they only saw them and welcomed them from a distance, admitting that they were foreigners and strangers on earth. People who say such things show that they are looking for a country of their own. If they had been thinking of the country they had left, they would have had opportunity to return. Instead, they were longing for a better country—a heavenly one. Therefore God is not ashamed to be called their God, for he has prepared a city for them.

JAMES 5:16

Therefore confess your sins to each other and pray for each other so that you may be healed. The prayer of a righteous person is powerful and effective.

1 PETER 5:6-7

Humble yourselves, therefore, under God's mighty hand, that he may lift you up in due time. Cast all your anxiety on him because he cares for you.

1 JOHN 5:11

And this is the testimony: God has given us eternal life, and this life is in his Son.

1 JOHN 5:13

I write these things to you who believe in the name of the Son of God so that you may know that you have eternal life.

REVELATION 1:17-18

When I saw him, I fell at his feet as though dead. Then he placed his right hand on me and said: "Do not be afraid. I am the First and the Last. I am the Living One; I was dead, and now look, I am alive for ever and ever! And I hold the keys of death and Hades…"

REVELATION 14:13

Then I heard a voice from heaven say, "Write this: Blessed are the dead who die in the Lord from now on."

"Yes," says the Spirit, "they will rest from their labor, for their deeds will follow them."

REVELATION 21:1-7

Then I saw "a new heaven and a new earth," for the first heaven and the first earth had passed away, and there was no longer any sea. I saw the Holy City, the new Jerusalem, coming down out of heaven from God, prepared as a bride beautifully dressed for her husband. And I heard a loud voice from the throne saying, "Look! God's dwelling place is now among the people, and he will dwell with them. They will be his people, and God himself will be with them and be their God. 'He will wipe every tear from their eyes. There will be no more death' or mourning or crying or pain, for the old order of things has passed away."

He who was seated on the throne said, "I am making everything new!" Then he said, "Write this down, for these words are trustworthy and true."

He said to me: "It is done. I am the Alpha and the Omega, the Beginning and the End. To the thirsty I will give water without cost from the spring of the water of life. Those who are victorious will inherit all this, and I will be their God and they will be my children.

ABOUT THE AUTHOR

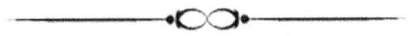

Lorinda Buckingham, Founder and CEO of Modern Empowerment, is a serial Entrepreneur, Business Strategist, Success Blueprint Developer, and Career Change Agent. She is best known for her down-to-earth, confident training style that delivers powerful principles in personal and professional development in leadership, business, and empowerment, that connects with diverse audiences to grow strong organizations and live their best lives. Lorinda's book—The Irreplaceable Mother—has touched the lives of many people. Lorinda's best selling audio series, The Modern Executive Success Blueprint 1.0 empowers individuals to step into their confidence, conquer their fears, uncover their passion, and more! The Modern Executive podcast is the ultimate leadership empowerment podcast heard on major podcast outlets such as iTunes, Google Play, and Alexa to empower contemporary leaders to live a life of freedom, balance, and faith for success in a contemporary world.

Lorinda has been successful in the corporate and business arenas and now shares her expertise with others through training, coaching, and speaking that empowers leaders to empower leadership in others. Her popular blog https://lorindabuckingham.com/blog reaches wide audiences. Lorinda's twitter account @Lori_Buckingham is known for sharing leadership, business, and inspirational tips. Lorinda is highly sought after for speaking, coaching, and training and can be booked at modernempowermentgroup@gmail.com or online at https://lorindabuckingham.com. Lorinda has turned her dream into a reality and would like to continue to share what she has learned in her quest for freedom, balance, and faith for success.

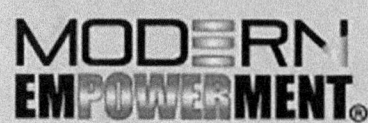 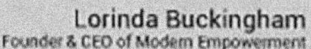 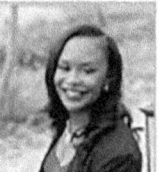

Develop Your Self.
Build Your Team.

WE ENHANCE, EQUIP & EMPOWER LEADERS TO EMPOWER LEADERSHIP IN OTHERS. OUR DEVELOPMENT TRAINING AND COACHING PROGRAMS GROW THE LEADERSHIP AND BUSINESS CAPABILITIES OF INDIVIDUALS, AND ALIGNS THEIR PERSONAL GROWTH WITH A BUSINESS STRATEGY. HERE IS HOW WE CAN HELP YOU:

 ASSESMENTS Receive valuable feedback that will impact your journey to become a highly effective leader including but not limited to DISC assessments, 360 Brand analysis, Youth DISC & Programs, Leadership Assessments, Success Blueprints, and more!

 TRAINING Become a better team leader or successful mentor by diving into our programs and specialized training.

 COACHING Connect with an experienced and certified personal and professional development coach who understand your challenges and support your growth.

 RESOURCES Equip yourself and your team with one of many resources that best fits your leadership interests. We seamlessly integrate into your regular operations with on-location, web-based, or streaming services. Our programs are flexible and affordable to fit most budgets.

 EVENTS Take your development to the next level at one of our Live Events, Mastermind Groups, or book us for your next event.

Lorinda Buckingham is the Founder and CEO of Modern Empowerment, LLC, and Certified Speaker, Trainer, Coach, DISC Specialist, Brand Specialist, and more! Connect with Lorinda today!

For more information on how we can serve you, visit WWW.LORINDABUCKINGHAM.COM. To read Lorinda's latest thoughts on leadership, visit WWW.LORINDABUCKINGHAM.COM /blog.

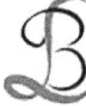 MODERN EMPOWERMENT. BUCKINGHAM
Freedom, Balance, and Faith for Success
Personal and Professional Development Training and Consulting Firm
Website: https://LorindaBuckingham.com
Email: ModernEmpowermentGroup@gmail.com

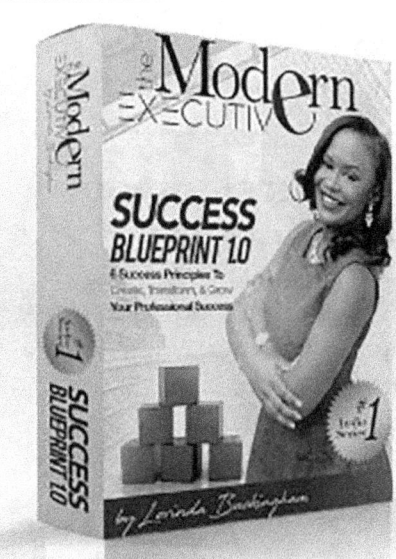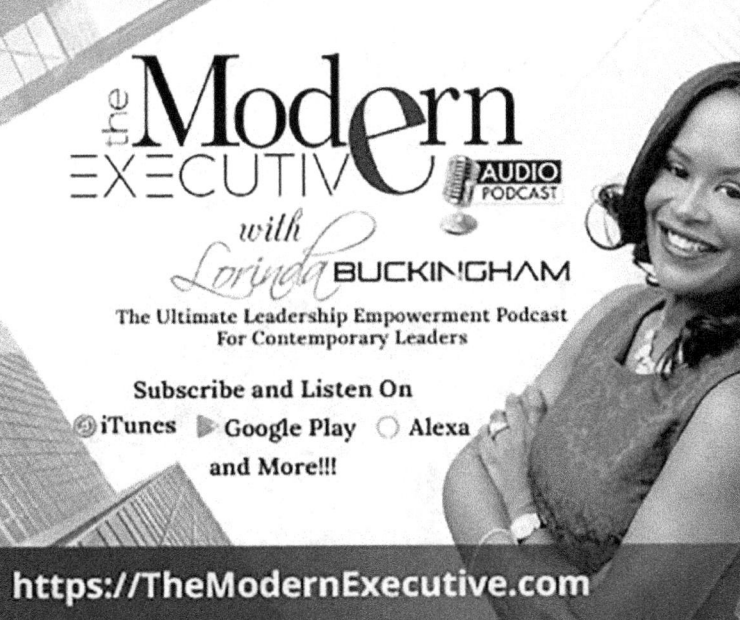

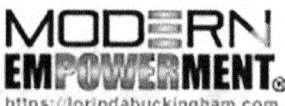
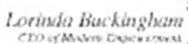

Overwhelmed With Understanding and Building Your Brand?

Get To Know The Brand—You! This Personal Branding program is the critical feedback you need to expand your life, career, and business.

ALIGNMENT 360°

Uncover your personal brand so that you can have insight into how others think about you. Discover your brand qualities to understand your professional reputation to enhance your career, grow your business, increase your influence, and much more! Get started today!
www.LorindaBuckingham.com

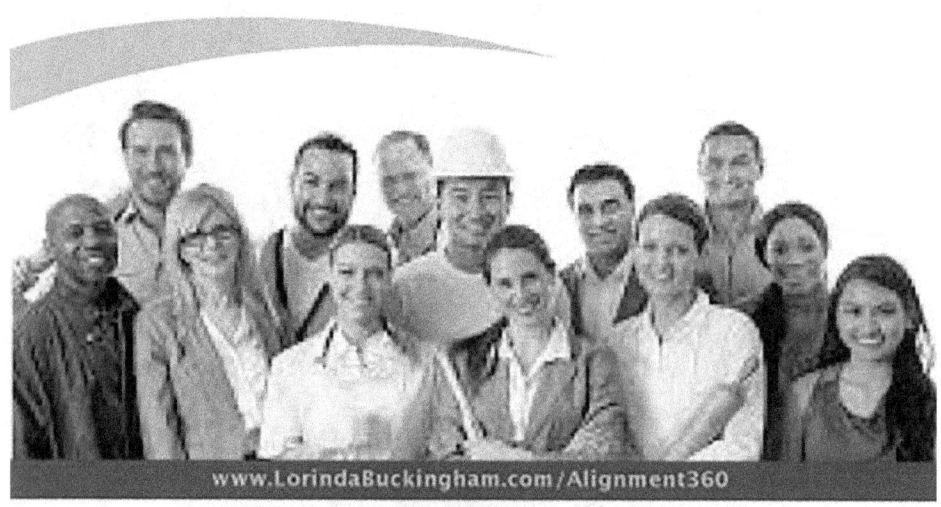

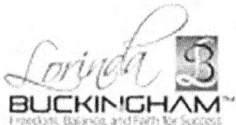

Lorinda Buckingham is *the Creator and Founder of Modern Empowerment, a Personal and Professional Development Training and Consulting firm. Lorinda is the host and teacher on The Modern Executive Podcast which is heard on major outlets, and creator of The Modern Executive Success Principles 1.0. She is a highly sought after Business Strategist, Success Blueprint Developer, Career Change Agent, and is a Certified Speaker, Trainer, Coach, and Brand Specialist. Lorinda looks forward to being able to add value to you, your team, or non-profit to grow leadership and business capabilities and to align personal development with a business strategy.*

To Work With Lorinda or Book Lorinda For Your Next Event,
Please Contact Us For Consultations And Bookings At
modernempowermentgroup@gmail.com

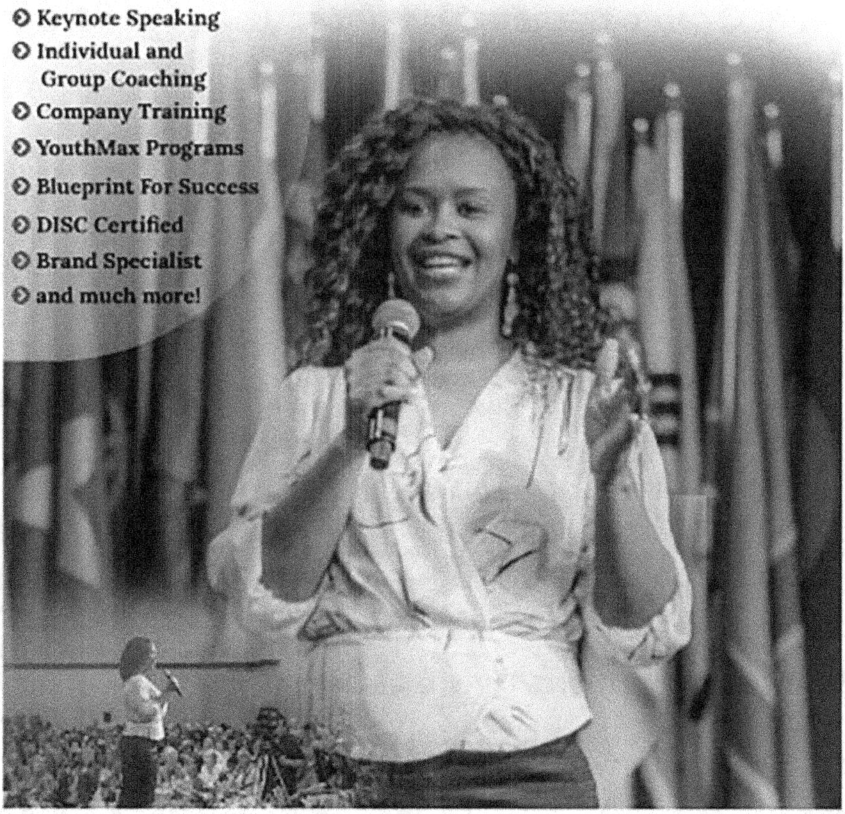

- Keynote Speaking
- Individual and Group Coaching
- Company Training
- YouthMax Programs
- Blueprint For Success
- DISC Certified
- Brand Specialist
- and much more!

MODERN EMPOWERMENT *Lorinda* BUCKINGHAM
Freedom, Balance, and Faith for Success
Personal and Professional Development Training and Consulting Firm
Website: https://LorindaBuckingham.com
email : ModernEmpowermentGroup@gmail.com

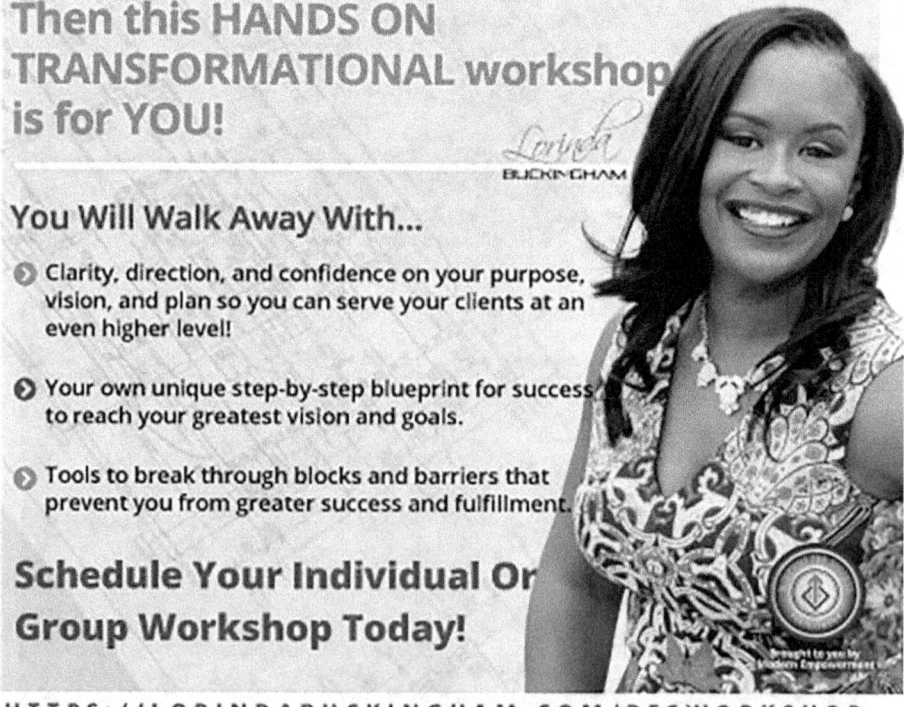

www.ingramcontent.com/pod-product-compliance
Lightning Source LLC
Chambersburg PA
CBHW071401290426
44108CB00014B/1642